# How to Create the Dental Practice of Your Dreams

## Guidelines to Achieving Joy and Success in Dentistry and Life

# How to Create the Dental Practice of Your Dreams

## Guidelines to Achieving Joy and Success in Dentistry and Life

John A. Wilde, D.D.S.

The Novel Pen
210 Windy Hills
Hamilton, Illinois 62341

First printing 1997

---

ISBN 0-9648511-8-0

LCCN 96-69301

---

Design and printing services provided by About Books, Inc., 425 Cedar Street, P.O. Box 1500, Buena Vista, CO 81211, (800) 548-1876.

# Dedication

This book has been written for my profession, as a small token of recompense for the gifts—material, intellectual and spiritual—with which dentistry has blessed me.

And to the young innocents who proudly join the ranks of dentistry each year. They are our future, and too little effort has been expended to acknowledge and nurture them. This work is my humble attempt to meet their needs and correct that injustice.

# Foreword

Too often in our professional lives we envy—then try to copy—many of the high profile dental practice management gurus on the lecture circuit. For many, this proves to be an exercise in futility, because we don't have the skills or charisma that they possess and then we feel bad when we can't do what they "claim to be doing."

It may come as a surprise to us that many of those we "idolize" aren't doing everything they claim to be doing either. In fact, they encounter the *same* stresses and problems that we do day to day . . . they just don't *admit* to having the frustrations of us average "dentists."

I guess that's why I like Dr. John Wilde so much. After reading his first book, *Bringing Your Practice Into Focus,* I thought . . . "Now here's a real guy—just like me—telling it the way it really is!" And here's a guy who has found a way to make it all work, obtain financial security, and retain his sanity in the process.

I finally had the pleasure of meeting John (in person) for breakfast at our "Fifth Annual $1,000,000 Spring Break Seminar" in Destin, Florida, in March 1996. He was just how I thought he would be. He's caring, honest, thought-provoking, and probably a lot like most of you reading this.

What makes John so special is that he's an average person who's found a way to achieve *above* average results. And that's what I like about him; he is doing something that every dentist can achieve, if they truly have the desire to do so.

It doesn't take extraordinary clinical skills, "Hollywood looks," or outstanding charisma to do what John is doing. His writing style is so easy to read and follow that almost anyone can achieve the results he talks about. His books "cookbook" the steps needed to achieve the results he's achieving.

Almost every day I receive a letter or telephone call from a 50+-year-old, burned-out dentist with *considerable* debt, no retirement plan in place, and no money to live on. It's sad, but it really doesn't have to be that way if we learn from those available to help us. Just ask John!

So sit back, relax, and learn from Dr. John Wilde. His latest book, *How to Create the Dental Practice of Your Dreams,* will help *you* develop the practice and life that *you* deserve.

**—Woody Oakes, D.D.S.**
**Editor of *The Profitable Dentist* Newsletter**

# Contents

# Introduction

CONGRATULATIONS! I assume all of the readers of this hopefully worthy tome have completed, or will soon complete, a doctorate level education. You are one of a **select few** who have completed 20 or more years of successful education—a DOCTOR.

For some reason, those who achieve such a gigantic accomplishment often take this honor rather lightly. Maybe the sheer length of time needed to realize this goal makes the actual fact of completion nothing more than another of what have been so many steps on a sometimes seemingly endless road. Perhaps you are too close to this great moment in your personal history to see it for the wonderful achievement it truly is.

(Maybe the fact that all of your classmates—many of whom you know to not be that bright—are doctors too, makes it hard to see this as a triumph. After all, how big a deal can graduating from dental school be if Fred made it?)

But it is necessary that you now take some time to glory in your achievement. I have many goals I wish to accomplish in the act of writing this book. (A guy has to have some dreams if he decides to spend almost two years to bring such a project to fruition!) Nothing is more central to my desires than demonstrating the essential need—superior to all other pursuits—of achieving a life filled with JOY! The teaching of this vital fact begins at this very moment.

A critical facet of this journey to joy is the ability to acknowledge the great moments, the true achievements in life, and take justifiable pride and satisfaction in that which you have earned.

CELEBRATE SUCCESS! I don't mean with some drunken pub crawl. Alcohol and drugs are great dangers—potential poisons—to all in the professions. Be as wary of them as you would be of venomous snakes. Maybe it's our relative wealth—our almost effortless ability to afford and obtain these crutches to life. Perhaps the stress all professionals deal with all of their lives makes us prone to the siren song of these vile tempters. Maybe it is simply hubris, the arrogance that lets us believe WE are too special to fall under their sway, that puts us at risk. Whatever the reasons, alcohol and other drugs are threats, both to the continuation of the degree we now celebrate and certainly to the joy we all seek.

The meaningful celebration of which I speak is accomplished quietly, internally. The drinking in, the savoring of a long and difficult task—a trail fraught with much pain and danger—that you have successfully completed. You're tired to the bone, bleeding, no doubt, from the cerebellum, but triumphant. **Feel the joy that true accomplishment brings!** This type of quiet, well-deserved satisfaction will last a lifetime, and unlike a party, will leave you with no regrets or pain in the morning.

But there is another danger at this moment of passage that we will touch on but lightly here. It is the development of a sense—an attitude—that by our efforts and achievements we have become better than others. What we have attained is great. Important. Significant. But not an event to sequester us from the rest of mankind. I believe the root of such feelings of superiority to be FEAR. And driven by inner fears, the great doctor flees from mankind by isolating herself from intimacy with others.

This fear, insecurity—call it what you will—holds a great danger. Another vital step in the road to joy is to see the oneness of all life, despite the many ways this essential fact is hidden from our eyes by life's many veils of illusion.

But we have plenty of time together to dwell on the sweet mystery of joy. Now is the time for celebration! Deep, sincere internal appreciation of the great deed you have performed. Please take a moment to reflect on the difficult passage of your years of formal education. The great quest for the holy grail of Doctor you have now, or soon will have, completed.

Feels good, doesn't it? And well it should.

Now that the formalities are over, and we have mutually savored your achievement, it's time to get on with our work. I reiterate my sincere desire that this book not merely help you achieve a level of success in your chosen profession of dentistry beyond your dreams, but also help steer you further along the pathway to a life filled with joy. Both of these goals, you must admit, are not meager ambitions.

How can these twin goals be realized? Any teacher, if he or she is to be successful, must be understood and believed as a person. To accept and thus trust someone, you must first know them. I realize, nothing is more boring than to be forced to listen to people talk at length about themselves! But in this case, for the bond of trust to develop that I feel is essential to the attainment of our goals, it is necessary.

Good news! The journey of my life that we will briefly peruse (recall if the description seems extensive, it took me 49 years and counting to live it) is akin to the path you have chosen. Its example may inspire or enlighten you. Or it may just leave you real achievers feeling superior! Whatever the final result, let us begin our time together with a review of the adventure that has been my life.

Okay, Lincoln has a better personal story. I wasn't born in a log cabin and never studied by candlelight. (Sneaking looks at *Playboy* under the covers with a flashlight is not an equivalent accomplishment.) But my beginning was humble enough. I was born December 14, 1946, in the little village of Lansing, Iowa, to become one of its 1,000 souls huddled along the banks of the great Mississippi River.

I was the firstborn of what was to become, over the course of fifteen years, a family of seven. Let me pause briefly on our journey here to give my condolences to the disproportionately many in the health professions who are firstborn. The helpers, the setters of positive example. It was not an easy lot we drew.

My dad, Mit Wilde, had returned from four-plus years of active duty in World War II to court and wed my mom, Jeanne Kehr Wilde, in a whirlwind romance. Dad entered college, but soon found out "little Johnny" was on the way. He withdrew from school and found a job. Dad's college career was ended in but a few weeks and he spent his years between then and retirement laboring—mostly in factories.

Mom had finished her degree in education during the war years, but in those enlightened days pregnant teachers weren't allowed in the classroom. Her teaching career suspended by the birth of five children, Mom worked at a variety of part-time jobs and raised our growing family, only returning to education when my baby brother Jerry was three, about the time I left for college.

My parents had no money to help finance my education, much as they wished to. But they had given me a great gift. I had always "known" I would go to college, and I had always "known" I would be personally responsible for the expense. My career in the labor force began officially at age 8 with a paper route. I can still recall holding out a handful of coins to let my customers select their own change. I couldn't do the math! (Not too much has changed in my math ability over the years, although I can now sure make change for a buck!)

Three years later, at the tender age of 11, I found full-time employment in a boat harbor located directly across from our home. I worked 7 days a week all summer long and weekends in the spring and fall. My starting salary was $.35 per hour. At 11 I may not have been worth that. I worked an average of 70 hours a week. Most summers I never took a day off.

After four years of employment at the marina, which saw my wages skyrocket to a heady $1.00 per hour, other jobs followed— in a hardware store owned by my grandfather, a sawmill, the local hayfields, factory work with my father. I cut grass, shoveled snow (lots of that in northernmost Iowa) and nailed together fish boxes as piecework. The net result was my having $3,000 in the bank when I entered the University of Iowa in 1964.

With the help of part-time school-year work and summer jobs, plus scholarships, I managed financially and my grades were good. I entered dental school in 1968. I married the love of my life, Joann, the summer after my freshman year in dental school. She had a year remaining to complete her degree in medical technology and I proudly (read stupidly) refused all generous offers of financial help from her parents. By the end of our first year of married bliss and my sophomore year in dental school, we were broke, but Jo had earned her degree and entered the work force, only to discover a month later that we were to become parents.

No money, no insurance. I took a night job as a campus policeman. Thus began a cycle of going to class my junior year from 8 a.m. to 5 p.m., studying, sleeping and eating until 10:30 p.m. when I reported for my night shift of "protecting the peace." Then home at 7 a.m. to shower and go back to school. On the good nights, when I had little homework, I slept 3 hours.

On March 13th, 1971 we had a son—John Jr. The doctor was immediately paid, and Jo and I were both pooped. Now—finally!— to my point. When I graduated from the University of Iowa College of Dentistry in 1972 we were a total of $3,000 in debt. I took a job working for a wonderful man, Dr. David Shaw in Cresco, Iowa, for the summer while waiting to enter the army in August of that year. I had been a student extern the summer before in Dr. Shaw's office, leaving Jo and baby Johnny in Iowa City for three months to live in Dave's home and work in his office, like a member of the family. I learned a great deal about the *practice* of dentistry that summer. When I left for military basic training in August, three months after my graduation, we had saved enough money to pay off the bills of our combined nine years of self-financed education.

I surely love protracted anecdotes that feature me as the heroic character. But the lengthy tale has this point, with direct bearing on our journey: to show it was and is possible to complete an education relatively free of debt. It was not easy. I often went two or three days without sleep. I don't want any of my four children to ever endure such hardships, yet it can be done.

But what if this information finds you too late? What if, like so many of your contemporaries, as you sit reading these words you are already deeply in debt? THE PRINCIPLES HOLD TRUE. They always do. The principle here is a commitment to struggling, sacrificing and doing without to EARN WHAT YOU RECEIVE. Not mortgaging your future by going into debt to enjoy the things you desire immediately. But rather choosing to wait, delaying gratification until by your efforts you have earned the possessions you wish for.

It is not too late to choose the path of hard and honest toil to earn what you possess. THIS PATH REQUIRES, AS A TOKEN FOR ADMISSION, MERELY THAT YOU MAKE THE *CHOICE* TO TAKE IT. We will discuss choices throughout the book. Can you understand your life to be nothing more than the sum of the decisions you have made?

In 1972, after our summer of running Dr. Shaw's practice while he vacationed in Europe, Jo, baby Johnny and I entered the U.S. Army Dental Corps. It was a great two years. I polished my neophyte dental skills and was honestly treated as an officer and gentleman. I studied the dental books I had slighted in honor of the excitement of a career in law and order (and the paycheck I received). Forty-hour weeks, or less, were as nothing to me—a veteran of years of 100-hour efforts. I read, exercised, caught up on parties for a year. Then my search for a practice location began in earnest.

I was stationed at Fort Lewis, Washington, near Seattle. Jo and I had decided to return to our native Iowa to live (which was, coincidentally, the only state in which I was licensed to practice!). I spent months writing, calling, investigating possible practice opportunities of every ilk. I also invested hours of study and talking to supply-house representatives about equipment and office design.

We took a great chunk of our meager financial resources—and we saved a goodly percentage of the roughly $16,000 per year that was my military salary—and flew our little family, now four in number with the addition of Heather Jean, back to Iowa. (We were poor, but prolific. Maybe that explains why "the poor are always with us.")

My mom and dad watched the little ones for two weeks, while Jo and I drove their car thousands of miles around the entire state examining the opportunities we had identified. A few months later, we again flew back and made a second two-week sojourn to closely study our final three choices, and selected Keokuk, Iowa, as the place we would begin our practice and make a home for our family.

This is another **KEY POINT**. The hours of research, the precious time and money that we spent on this vital decision—almost a year-long effort that consumed a great deal of our savings—led to our eventual early success in practice. Once again, hard work and personal sacrifice were the keys. (I am a master at the long cut, the hard way to a destination.) We'll discuss the details of selecting an ideal practice location at great length shortly, but the skill, exertion and desire we exhibited in our efforts to find the right place is what I'd like you to focus on now.

How did we know what to look for? By reading, talking and concentrating our total awareness on the problem before us. Could we "afford" to use our entire military paid leave time and much of our savings on this quest? So much of success is determined by what things are seen as expenses and which are viewed as investments. Our search clearly was an investment in the future of our lives. *No single factor has been as significant in our success as our initial choice of a practice location.*

What in the world did we spend all that time discovering in Keokuk, Iowa, that was of such value? A hoard of buried treasure? In a manner, yes. We found that we liked the town—13,000 was a nice-sized community for my country-raised wife and her small-town husband. I liked the Mississippi that flowed hard on the town's edge and the recently constructed YMCA. Jo liked the new mall. The schools seemed good, and the people were unfailingly Midwest-friendly. The river setting, many parks and the beauty of the area combined to create a community that we found very desirable to live in. We were also within a five-hour drive of our Iowa family.

Be certain that the community you choose in which to practice is one you will be happy living in. My first associate was from the big city. He was a great guy, a good dentist and did extremely well in our office, but after one year moved with his homesick wife back to the city area and family they had left. Being "successful" but unhappy is definitely not what this book is about.

In the search for our future home we also talked with local dentists. They were all very busy, and the majority of them would never see age 60 again. We believed the relatively advanced age of the local practitioners to be an important consideration for our professional future. With one exception, they all felt our office would be successful at once and would gladly refer patients to us. The only specialist in the area, an orthodontist, actively recruited us. The bankers were friendly and willing to assist us with financing. This had not been the case in every town we evaluated. I identified a possible office location that I liked and worked out a tentative lease agreement.

We had every assurance we would be busy and were treated very well by the area dentists and other professionals. On our second trip, we finalized the office lease, reached an agreement with a bank, and found an apartment to rent. We were set.

On August 17, 1974, we first opened the office doors to patients. It had taken us two months after leaving the army to complete the construction of the office. The portion of the existing building where my office was to be located featured dirt floors when we first set eyes on it. I very carefully hired two staff members (interviewing candidates in the only available space, our tiny apartment's bedroom) and spent hours creating an office policy manual—a vital aid to practice management that in a revised form still serves us today.

But here is an amazing thing. We didn't as yet have our office or home number in the phone book, yet the first day the office was finally complete enough to see patients, we were already booked several weeks in advance. Mostly referred by other dentists, and good old word of mouth, patients had called our apartment to schedule office visits. This running start was the first fruits of the year-long labor to find the right location for an office.

The office I built had two completely equipped operatories and was designed, wired and plumbed for a third. The total investment for equipment, supplies, leasehold improvements came to $30,000. I had a bank waiting and willing to loan us money when we discovered our exact capital needs. The loan was never made.

We had arrived in Keokuk with $10,000 in savings, from our months working with Dr. Shaw and our two years in the army. My beloved Grandpa Kehr had loaned us $10,000 of his very hard-earned hardware store money. As the bills slowly trickled in, we generated the remainder of the needed funds from the practice's cash flow. We lived in an upstairs two-bedroom apartment two blocks from my office and survived on very little. In March of 1975, **seven months** after we first opened the office door, a very proud and not nearly grateful enough grandson repaid the $10,000 he owed his grandfather. We owned our office, "free of all debt." (A phrase that I never tire of hearing!)

How significant a difference this freedom from debt has made in our financial condition over the years is difficult to calculate. IMMENSE is a gross understatement. I don't even care to reflect on how much the typical 15 years of debt repayment for an office loan would have delayed our reaching financial freedom. How was the attainment of a debt-free office achieved in seven months? By a combination of careful planning, great effort, and NOT SPENDING MONEY WE HADN'T TRULY EARNED.

I won't bore you much longer (I hope!). Our office paid for, we bought the home we still live in today and moved in on May 31, 1975. With a steady and rising income from the practice, we knew we could afford the newly constructed country home our little family wanted. We paid for the home within three years. By age 40—after thirteen years in private practice—I had enough money saved and invested that I no longer needed to work. I still chose to treat patients, but even in 1986 our income from investments exceeded $80,000 per year. With no debt, and our simple choice of lifestyle, that was money enough.

We'll touch on parts of my story, the only life I truly know, as we progress on our journey. I hope you've already clearly identified some of the keys to my success. Sadly, they don't include a brilliant mind, gifted hands, great looks or an outgoing, lovable personality. They are composed of the much less exciting gifts—the ability to set a goal, hold it clearly in sight and then work like a dog to achieve it. I wish I knew an easier way.

Let me introduce a last bit of information that may further help you to trust and believe what I tell you. Allow me to enumerate the reasons I believe I am qualified to undertake the daunting task of advising another human being as to how to proceed with your career and life:

1. As you've seen from our discussion to date, I've lived it. I believe many of my readers also wish to attain financial success. I think all seek counsel on how to fill their existence with joy. I'll share my journey with unblinking honesty—the good, bad and ugly—with every reader.

2. I taught at the University of Iowa, senior dental student clinic, in 1974. I enjoyed the experience greatly, but the two-hour drive and pressures of an amazingly quickly growing practice forced me to abandon the task. Yet, I have experienced dental education from the status of both student and instructor.

3. I have had five dental student externs grace my office for five- to six-week periods, as I spent my summers with Dr. Shaw. I have enjoyed these young people's stays with us tremendously and have been honored to act as their mentor. I was shocked and saddened when the Iowa College of Dentistry abandoned this worthy program, terminating the one chance students had to learn the real profession of dentistry (as opposed to the artificial world of dental school). Ending this beneficial program is inexplicable to me and can be only comprehensible from the rarefied air of academia, so separated from the mundane life of other mere mortals.
4. I have a son and daughter who are both finishing graduate-level educations. "Little Johnny"—all 200 pounds of him—has graduated from Southern Illinois College of Law. Baby Heather completed at least her first graduate degree in finance at the same time. I have their contemporary educational experiences, quite different from my own, to draw upon.
5. I have employed five associates in my office over the years. I know a great deal of what the senior dentists who seek associates quest for, as well as how this delicate relationship works—or fails to work. We will discuss at length what a potential associate should look for in a prospective place of employment, as well as examining what traits the senior dentist might admire.
6. I have started an office, and seen it grow to a group of three doctors we currently enjoy. I will be glad to share what I have learned, pro or con, from all of the configurations of dental practice I've personally experienced.
7. I like to write! As of this date, I've had approximately 30 magazine articles and three books published—two dental and one fiction. I only began writing in 1992. It gives me something to do.

But the above enumerated points are mere facts. The main quality that I feel makes me a legitimate choice to serve as your mentor is compassion. I find the work of dentistry to be very difficult. In 1994 I only saw patients on 70 days. If the clinical practice of dentistry contained great joy for me, I would have drunk much more deeply from its waters (70 days a year is barely sipping!). As I have detailed, the eight years of self-financed college was like a survival course, which I passed by the slimmest of margins. Truly, I have felt your pain.

Also, as a result of my writing I have occasion to speak to many in our fine profession, as I include my home phone number in every published work. A great number of these doctors are very dissatisfied with the business of dentistry—some distressed to the point of being frightening to me. A goodly percent of these intensely unhappy people have practices that would be deemed successful by most criteria. To see them this disenchanted is scary! Where is the joy?

Let's proceed from this introduction to peruse two areas you must comprehend if you desire to know, understand and believe me. First, we'll take a brief look at my dental practice as it exists today. Then we'll begin our study of the attainment of joy. This bifurcated vision will reveal to you a great deal about who I am, what I've done, and in what I believe. It will also establish a firm foundation from which to begin your professional and personal journey.

I assure you, we'll get to how many handpieces you should order and what is the ideal office floor-covering, but we won't build our dental house on sand. We'll begin by studying a method by which you can grow as a person and create a foundation of bedrock upon which your practice and life can be securely based.

## Chapter One

# The Subject Was Joy

Allow me to begin this discussion with the acknowledgment of a powerful and amazing book entitled *The Evolving Self* (hereafter *Self*), written by Mihaly Csikszentmihalyi.

There is an ancient saying that when the student is ready, a teacher will appear. As I read *Self*, I felt the book had been written just for me. No work could have more closely fitted the exact mental state I was in at the time I read those words, or more precisely satisfied my intellectual needs. I would be delighted if even a handful of readers were so affected by my words.

I cannot reproduce all of the richness and wonder of this great book here. Of course, I highly recommend it to all of you and wish to thank my friend, Dr. Morton Ehudin, who brought the book to my attention.

In this chapter I will borrow generously from the book's espoused tenets to buttress my personal beliefs more fully. I'll also attempt to customize *Self's* wisdom specifically for this audience by applying its concepts to both personal and dental situations with which we're all, or soon will be, intimately familiar.

The material occupies the prominent position of Chapter One in this book for the following reasons:

1. The information, though challenging to comprehend, once grasped is wonderfully exciting. It has the ability to release the energy needed to propel the reader on a journey of personal understanding and self-discovery that is essential if this book's objectives are to be achieved.

   I know, this is a dental book. But no single ingredient is more vital to the success of any venture than the central figure in the enterprise—in this case you, doctor—being clearly focused and **energized** toward the attainment of carefully set goals.

2. I want each reader to understand who I am and believe it best to begin this process with a study of my deeply held personal beliefs. In this chapter, as well as in the ones which follow, we'll explore in depth my professional history and the theories that lead to whatever success I can lay claim to in that realm, but more essential than a mere history of my actions is a comprehension of the personal beliefs that motivated my every deed.

3. My readers' PERSONAL JOURNEY TO JOY is of paramount importance to me. Understanding this material is foundational to the attainment of joy.

I must beg the indulgence and effort of my audience here. The concepts that make up this chapter are admittedly difficult and complex. They are also ABSOLUTELY CENTRAL to the meaning of this book. Please take your time and understand this vital information before going on with your reading. Believe me, the following information is an essential segment of our journey to joy.

It is one of my foundational personal beliefs that our **every thought and action is driven by a single impulse: We BELIEVE the ultimate fruit of our activity will be JOY.** The form of this joy we seek varies from time to time, from person to person. It may be wealth, health, success, popularity, finding the right mate or performing well in the sport of your choosing . . . but our quest to attain happiness, however its form may currently be perceived, is the never-ending motivation for all that we do.

It is sadly true that even our mightiest efforts often fail to produce the fruits of joy we seek. For many practicing dentists, the years of education and the effort required to create and continue their practice have not resulted in the rewards they had anticipated or at least desired. In a similar fashion, the "joy" of drug use soon turns into the bitter dregs of pain for the users—yet the motive behind our career paths, as well as the reason for taking drugs, was certainly the desire to attain joy.

One of the myriad ways we vary as individuals is in what possessions and actions we believe will lead us to happiness. For any given one of us the pathway may seem to be attaining money, a great car, a "trophy" spouse, or dwelling in a hilltop mansion. Yet despite these individual variations, all of us are guided in our quest for personal joy by the same three basic forces. If we are to be free to select a lifestyle based on personal choice, it is imperative that we understand these primary motivational dynamics in our lives.

## 1. Genetics

With our background as scientists, this particular drive may be the most meaningful to us, and I believe it to be the most compelling of the three forces.

We all have, encoded in our very DNA, the timeless message that we must make every effort consistent with the continuation of our own lives and the reproduction of our species. This is our genetic imperative! Were it not so, the human species would have fallen victim to the merciless realities of evolution many millennia ago. This directive is vital to our continued existence both as individuals and as a species.

It is to satisfy this innate drive that we accumulate personal power—be it in the form of food, money, possessions, shelter or even **years of education**. With each of these objects obtained, our chances for survival are enhanced. (I believe the genetic demand to reproduce has caused enough well-documented problems since the times of the siege of Troy to require no further embellishment from me.)

But a part of this genetic coding to survive is a pre-disposition of our minds, when unoccupied, to be eternally vigilant (and thus eternally restless) in an effort to discover and develop new and better strategies to enhance both our own and our species' odds for survival.

This bias, built into our very beings with the most noble of motives—the continuation of the individual and thus the species—places us on a mental treadmill that knows no limitations. It is the nature of the human mind, when left unabated, to move ever closer to feelings of fear, anger, depression and jealousy. This recurring message of the mind could perhaps be best summarized as many variations of the basic theme "I WANT!".

The ancient tale of the fisherman, his catch—a magic flounder—and his never-satisfied wife who continually wanted more, has illustrated through the ages the perpetual dissatisfaction that is a part of humankind's nature.

This part of our inherent nature, when seen as a mechanism for enhancing our chances of survival, can be appreciated. But in our current times, freed from the great majority of acute risks to our lives, this eternal vigilance can become a negative factor. This very penchant for continuous improvement of our personal and species viability destroys that which we moderns so deeply crave: peace of mind.

Simply understanding the organic reality of this situation has been helpful to me. (At least I know I'm not the only one so afflicted.) We will discuss methods whereby we can partially control and channel these undeniable forces shortly. Awareness of their presence and power allows us to freely decide if we choose to follow their directives, or override them by decisions based on our own clear values. Briefly, we have the options to:

a) Involve ourselves with tasks to occupy and still our minds.

b) Develop skills to control our mental process using methods like meditation. I have meditated for years with very positive and enjoyable effects, but—while I would recommend this activity to every reader—details of meditative techniques are beyond the scope of this book.

c) Or deliberately and carefully craft a meaningful life philosophy, a process we will deal with at great length within this text.

## 2. Cultural

Just as we are driven by genetically coded messages, we are also under the auspices of cultural imperatives. Summarized, these messages, internalized by each of us from infancy, all say that "our culture is the center of the universe." These beliefs provide us with an enhanced sense of importance and meaning. (And for Americans, when combined with military might, they may explain why we feel it acceptable to attack any third world power who doesn't agree with our ideas, ideals or outright demands.)

The strengthening of our culture enhances our chances of survival and thus is consistent with the biological and genetic messages we've just discussed.

The negative of culture's bidding is that if we blindly accept its messages, we forfeit our right to free choice. The gifts of any culture are great. They include our language, traditions and sense of stability. Certainly they shouldn't be abandoned. But every situation life presents us with should be scrutinized and understood on our own *clarified personal values level,* before we make decisions based on nothing more than cultural directives. (Starting a war keeps coming to mind.)

## 3. Sense of Selfhood

Man is the only creature with self-reflective consciousness. (i.e. We can think about ourselves.) I'll leave it to you gentle readers to label this ability as: A) a blessing, B) a curse, or most possibly C) both of the above.

This self-thought creates what we call our EGO or sense of ourself as a unique entity. The goal of the ego is to protect itself at all costs. But the ego encompasses not only who we are, (the biological organism itself) but also those we care about and for, as well as our valued possessions and rights.

With the development of ego, "good" becomes all things that enhance ourselves. "Bad" becomes all things which threaten this extended definition of self. This concept explains why someone who loses all her money might choose to take her life. Such persons don't decide to labor and earn more money, but instead select suicide, as if the money they lost had become an integral part of their self-identity.

The point of discussing all three of the above forces is to illustrate that the decisions we make are usually not completely of our own volition, but are greatly—yet subtly—influenced by the above-named sources. To control our lives and develop consistent joy we must find a way to **self-develop** the rules we decide to live by, aware of and thus freed of these strong but subconscious forces that, unless controlled by our own will, tend to guide our decisions for us.

There is no point during the course of an individual's existence when the need to self-develop an environment totally consistent with his or her own true beliefs is more essential, or more possible, than when undertaking the creation of a professional vehicle—your practice—that will greatly impact your chances of attaining joy in your lifetime. A failure to be aware of the needs to:

a) Understand your own values clearly, and thus be able to

b) Create an environment where the unique YOU can find joy

can result in a practice built with the best intentions and greatest labors, that in no way accurately reflects what you personally believe.

A lack of self-reflection, and the insecurity that results when our values are imprecise, lead to attempts to create EVERYONE ELSE'S dental office. One must work to clarify personal beliefs and think deeply as to what leads to personal joy. This process will allow a philosophy to develop around which a practice that is consistent with your values—and thus can lead to joy—will be built. BEWARE of a failure in this basic premise that I believe accounts for so many in our profession surviving at an emotional level near despair.

As we briefly mentioned, there are pathways available that will allow us to develop this lifestyle of choice. One involves the activities we are involved in, while another deals with the development of our own unique mind-set.

The idea of FLOW in activities is probably familiar to most of you. There are times when we become so involved in what we are doing as to lose all sense of time and place. We are so engrossed in our pastime of the moment that the rest of the world seems to fall by the wayside.

I have frequently experienced flow while playing tennis, hunting or as I'm jogging. I often experience it when I write. The pleasantness of the flow sensation explains why such activities are among my favorite pastimes. Let me briefly sketch what is involved in the "flow" process:

1. Our attention narrows to some ***clearly defined goal*** with a manageable set of rules. (Such as hit the ball, or complete the chapter.)
2. We receive ***immediate feedback*** from our activity. (The tennis ball lands in the other court, or "beautiful words" fill the pages.)
3. THE CHALLENGES ARE IN BALANCE WITH OUR SKILL LEVELS. The capitals indicate my belief in the critical nature of this particular ingredient. Neither winning nor losing a tennis match 6-0 results in flow. Likewise, helping my son with a law school paper (which I know little about) or assisting my sixth grader on a writing assignment are both usually nonflow experiences, due to the imbalance of skill and challenges inherent in each situation.
4. Our clear goals allow ***total concentration***.
5. Our ***actions and awareness merge*** as one.

6. A *sense of control* is possible, but not easy. (I can hit the ball wherever I want, or I know exactly how I wish to express myself, but I must continue to focus or I will lose these marvelous gifts.)
7. We ***lose our sense of consciousness*** and become part of a greater entity. (The ball seems to seek the right place of its own volition, or the perfect words leap forth by themselves with me struggling mightily just to record them quickly enough.)
8. We have a ***totally altered sense of time***. (I am amazed when the match is over, or I glance up from the computer, completely unaware I've been writing for an hour past my normal lunch time.)

Flow is a wonderfully pleasant way to spend time. The more you can be involved in activities that create this experience, the happier you will become! While awareness of flow can change our behavior patterns by causing us to seek out such interests, none of us can live a life filled with nothing but continuous flow experiences. I doubt we'd have the strength, even if we had the opportunity. Yet we can develop our expertise at identifying situations that create flow in our lives and deliberately choose to become more involved in such activities.

For example, it is vital to the financial survival of any dental practice that the doctor be dedicated to the business aspect of the practice. These tasks may be intensely boring—such as poring over accountant reports. Often the business details are distressing, such as having to confront staff members for not performing their duty, or dealing with an unhappy patient. But if, as most professionals do, we consider financial well-being an essential ingredient to joy, we must pay the price of dealing with the realities of business if we hope to achieve success.

The same disciplines are essential for nonprofessional achievement. Overeating, failing to exercise, smoking or excessive drinking may all be "fun" to do, but few would argue that the net result of the aforenamed behavior is joy. Do you see that the choice to fill your life with nothing but "fun" activity isn't realistic and is not a viable pathway to joy?

It is self-evident how identifying and pursuing flow activities will enhance our personal time. There are viable alternatives to television and booze. But let me relate the concept of flow to our profession. If an activity is a great challenge and our skills are low in that area, we have **anxiety**. A great deal of dentistry still presents a challenge beyond my skills. After 26 years, the challenge is seldom the complexity of the procedure (I can always choose to refer or not treat), but more often deals with the unique difficulties of the patients themselves. Treating an upper second molar on a grossly obese patient with a strong gag reflex (is it redundant to add they are extremely apprehensive?) really tests my deodorant. WHEN OUR SKILLS ARE NOT UP TO THE CHALLENGE, OR IT IS OUR PERCEPTION THAT THEY AREN'T, WE FEEL ANXIETY.

When the challenge is low, and our skills are high, the result is **boredom**. Recall examinations on patients I've treated for years fall short of a ski trip to the Alps in regard to inherent excitement or joy.

It seems, in my professional life, that these two ingredients, anxiety and boredom, comprise most of my day. The great majority of the dental tasks I'm asked to accomplish I can do in my sleep! BORING. The rest of my activities involve things like performing a pulpotomy on a hot tooth for a patient I've never seen before who is scared to death. Do I have adequate skills to meet this challenge? Sometimes.

Early in my dental career, I got a pleasant sense of achievement from seating a crown with good margins, or even from placing a simple restoration correctly. Now my skills are to the point where, after 10,000 repetitions of the above, the only choices I have are boredom (all went well, as it always should) or anxiety (why the heck can't I get good anesthesia?).

The progression you'll see as your careers advance is from a preponderance of anxiety in the early years, where as yet immature skills are frequently tested, to an increase in boredom as routine duties take up more of your day. Both emotions are much less enjoyable than flow experiences, but there is no question that anxiety is considerably more unpleasant and unhealthy.

While I've never seen it described in just this manner, the foregoing scenario seems very similar to the dreaded "**burnout**" that is so ubiquitous in our profession. What's a poor dentist to do? We can make an effort to do more of the clinical procedures that are exciting and rewarding for us (flow opportunities) and elect to avoid those tasks that lead to boredom or anxiety. I wish you all great luck in this quest, but realistically, eliminating boredom and anxiety appears fairly hopeless within the practice of dentistry as I know it. (Which pretty well explains why I'm sitting here writing, rather than selecting the more lucrative choice of cutting precise holes in someone's molar.)

The second method available to free us from the grip of forces that control us, and thus place us foursquare on the pathway to joy, is to develop a **mental philosophy** that is consistent with the maximum attainment of joy.

Maybe—just maybe—it is possible to achieve joy within our profession from the context of helping others or from the awareness we are improving the quality of our patients' lives by the care we deliver. Or the work itself may remain a mixture of boredom and anxiety, but you find enjoyment from being with staff and patients. Perhaps you can derive satisfaction from being able to provide for the material needs of yourself and your family.

My point is that while it may be nearly impossible for most of us spit-soaked veterans to create an office where every day is a continual flow experience, free of anxiety and boredom, we could increase our personal joy through a change in our **perception** of the labors we perform.

I realize that in the early years of your career, merely surviving, emotionally and financially, is reason to rejoice. But the problems we are discussing will surely and negatively affect your life. It is so much easier to avoid a problem than to correct it. Ask any smoker. I hope my words can help guide you beginning practitioners towards a path of joy early in your journey, and save you many painful false steps.

Please take some deep breaths and refocus your powers of concentration. We've covered a lot of vital information already, but more essential and challenging data follows. Now that you're refocused, allow me to introduce two less than subtle clues to our desired intellectual destination in the form of the following quotations:

Sophocles: "**Wisdom** is the supreme part of **happiness**."

Montaigne: "The most manifest sign of **wisdom** is continual **cheerfulness**."

Please recall, our subject is joy (or happiness or cheerfulness or peace of mind) and we find it linked here inextricably with wisdom. If this is the case, we had better direct our efforts to a better understanding of this "wisdom thing."

There are three basic aspects of wisdom. Understanding this information is essential to the achievement of joy in any facet of our lives:

1. There are COGNITIVE SKILLS. This is a way of ***knowing***, or the process of collecting information—the learning of facts. Still so close to your years of formal educational experience, most of my readers will excel at this endeavor.
2. VIRTUE is a part of wisdom and is defined as a way of ***acting*** that is socially desirable. To know what to do (cognitive) but not to do it (by virtuous action) contains no wisdom. Neither does acting in a way inconsistent with our knowledge of reality.
3. Wisdom involves PERSONAL GOALS that lead to inner security and enjoyment. For example, actions that aren't consistent with our true values and don't result in the attainment of our goal and the resultant ***joy and peace*** are not wise.

Wisdom then is not mere knowledge. There are three factors that clearly differentiate the two:

1. Wisdom deals not with superficial experience, but with UNIVERSAL TRUTHS.
2. Wisdom isn't just awareness, but VIRTUOUS ACTION based on knowledge.
3. WISDOM ACTED ON FEELS GOOD. Thus we can use pain as a sure guide to alert us that our actions **are not wise.**

**WISDOM is KNOWLEDGE that is ACTED UPON to produce JOY.**

For so common a word and one as oft spoken (if seldom exhibited) as is "wisdom," it's surprising how little we know of the subject. Ask a few people you know and respect what "wisdom" is and I think you'll be surprised at the diversity and confusion in the answers you'll receive.

Let's now examine how we may obtain wisdom—a commodity that can't be bought, but must be earned. Allow me to suggest that wisdom is obtained by an increase in **complexity** in any given system. For purposes of illustration, those of you already in private practice, take a moment and mentally review the history of your own office collection policies over the years. See if you can appreciate the expansion of complexity as your system has evolved.

Complexity is derived from two diverse but interrelated sources. Increased complexity means an increase in **differentiation**. This means an increase in the number of parts of differing structure in any given system. In your collection procedures, differentiation could mean more written guidelines, more people and/or more time committed to your collection system or possibly adding a computer to assist your efforts.

An expansion in complexity also requires greater **integration**. This is the ability of different parts to **work together** to achieve a common goal.

For wisdom to result, our complexity increase must include BOTH an increase in differentiation (more and more parts added to the system) and also an advanced level of integration of these parts. If the differing parts don't work TOGETHER we have anything but wisdom and joy as a result.

This brings us to the enemy of wisdom and thus ultimately of joy: ENTROPY. You may recall the Second Law of Thermodynamics from your studies. This states that systems tend to return to randomness—for most of us our collection systems will illustrate this concept perfectly!

(A much less well-known word is NEGENTROPY which is the tendency for order to increase in a system. I assume we dentists haven't heard much of this as it damn near never occurs in our profession!)

There have been many "continuing education systems" around over the years that knew about the Second Law of Thermodynamics. For a fee, usually in the $20,000 range (this is powerful stuff!), they would explain the concept to you. In only a few months they could help you *set up office systems* and *install monitors* to continually evaluate the in-place systems. By using a monitoring process you were guarding against entropy, or the return toward the randomness that had previously afflicted you.

By sharing this information with you, I've already saved you $20,000, plus weeks of hanging around with these "second law" folks. If any of you feel overwhelmed by gratitude, you may make the check out to John A. Wilde for whatever part of the $20,000 your conscience dictates and consider yourself caught up on thermodynamics.

All of this theory is fine, necessary for your own understanding and increasing complexity—right? But if you can't find a way for this information to be applied immediately to improve your life, it's useless by my lights. So let's take a look at some examples in both our dental office and life in general where the concepts we've just discussed lead us to our goal of JOY.

In office, let's stick with collection policy as a topic we've all had, or will have, troubles with at times. Our precise definition of joy here is to collect 98% or more of production so:

a) We don't have unhappy clients who must be called by unhappy staff to ask them to pay their bill.

b) We don't have to endure the headaches of a "bite that was never right." (This occlusal problem is typically identified by the patient one year after the crown was seated and a day after the account was turned over for collection.)

c) We receive our just and due monetary rewards!

We attack this problem by *adding complexity*. Perhaps a staff meeting is held and office collection policies clearly outlined. These guidelines are written down and maybe even mailed to all our patients. The new policies are the *differentiation*. The *integration* includes having all the staff working together to give the same answers to patient questions and presenting a united front as regards office financial policy. (We'll deal extensively with team building and how essential it is to happiness and success in later chapters.)

In two months collections are 105%! Everybody is happy and you take the staff out for a celebratory dinner. One less problem in the world to worry about, because this one is solved, baby! You and your staff are wise and the knowledge of your collective wisdom (and the cash in the bank) fills you with joy.

Two years later collections are at 90%!!! You and your staff discuss this together—you purveyors of wisdom. Decay has set into the system. The Second Law of Thermodynamics has snuck up on your entire office and given it a Big Moose Hickey. You discover that if you currently have a collection system at all, it is random. You guess that when your receptionist Suzy left, all the trouble started. But you thought the problem was dealt with forever!

Again, the system is examined and possibly more complexity added. This time (after reading this book) you monitor the major parts of the system you and your staff co-develop and have one staff member personally responsible for each component. Over the years, you continue monitoring every month and your collection rate remains high. You even refine the system a bit as the years go by. This is the wisdom, with entropy's pernicious effect factored in, that leads to real joy.

As a personal example, let's say your jeans have become tight—a not uncommon problem for people confined to a desk or dental chair. You doubt every pair of pants could have shrunk. Time to take off some weight. You develop a diet plan and it's working, until two weeks pass, when you slip just a bit and doughnuts and entropy hit you with a double whammy that leaves you a corpulent, quivering mass.

The only answer to diets that work (this advice is complimentary) is an increase in wisdom. Your diet system grows more complex as you study good nutrition, exercise wisely and slowly work the weight down. As fruits replace potato chips, wisdom will be in the true change in the way you see yourself—as a slender, healthy, well-conditioned person.

To summarize, we all wish for joy. We must be aware of the subconscious forces of genetics, culture and ego that tend to rule our decision-making process. If we fail to be aware of their power, it will interfere with our ability to make individual decisions that are consistent with our own best interests and clear personal values.

We also need to comprehend that the human mind, when unoccupied by some labors, tends to restlessness. We can decrease the ill effects of said restlessness by identifying and engaging our mental processes in flow activities. Learning such skills as meditation can enhance peace of mind. But the real key—and a central focus of this book—will be the development of a personal and professional philosophy based on an understanding of wisdom, and thus on guard against entropy, that will yield a life filled with ***JOY!***

We must constantly evaluate our lives to see if we act with wisdom. Are our judgments based on accurate knowledge? Do we take action based on this awareness? And do these actions result in JOY? Let's look at one final example:

Do we have the knowledge that all mankind are special creatures, valuable in their own right? Without this awareness—*with wrong knowledge*—we will be in constant conflict and contention with our fellow man and thus continually lack peace of mind.

Or maybe we honor mankind in our mind, but tend to treat people in a negative, judgmental manner. The fruit of this *wrong action* will be pain that, when examined, can re-guide us back to the pathway to joy.

Examine everything in your life that causes pain and identify why that course of behavior is lacking in wisdom. Some painful actions may be based on biases you have held all of your life. IF THEY CAUSE YOU PAIN THEY ARE NOT WISE, no matter how your brilliantly rationalizing mind tries to convince you that THE OTHERS are wrong and you are right. The point isn't who's "right," whatever "right" is—but rather to be happy.

For you parents, how do YOU feel when you criticize and discipline your children? Sad? Upset? But you do it for their own good, right? What if you had the knowledge to chastise or direct in complete acceptance and love? If you acted based on this awareness, how would you then feel? How can this change come about in your life? How would this mind-set affect your relationship with your family, staff, friends and patients? Can you sense the aroma of the fruit that is wisdom?

I know this chapter was a somewhat tough—and dry—bolus to swallow. But I am blessed with readers who are among the most educated individuals in the history of the world! They are more than able to digest even this difficult fare. (At least I, as a dental student, was forced to read material much more challenging than this, and infinitely more boring!) Take a moment to review this information before going on to the more "fun stuff." The knowledge contained here has the potential to change every facet of your life in a most basic and profound manner.

We are moving next to a specific, fact-centered look at my dental practice and the philosophies behind it. Please hold every statement I make up to the criteria of wisdom and joy we have just discussed. Remember that nothing I say can have value unless it leads you to greater joy.

## Chapter Two

# The $2,000-Per-Day Net Practice

We have begun to examine some of my most deeply held beliefs. I hope, even at this early point in your careers, you can begin to see that all your strivings—from Little League to dental school completion—have been dedicated to the pursuit of joy.

Why did you wish to excel at sports, music or in school? Why is there a "special person" so vital to you? Why do you so desperately desire to excel both professionally and financially? These, as well as every other question central to your emotional well-being, are answerable by the same response: To make me happy!

Yet we are seldom consciously aware of this fact. And our unawareness often results in pain. I well recall the **desperation and terror** involved in beginning my dental practice. I can recollect no awareness in any part of my being that my struggles were motivated by a wish for happiness. Now, in retrospect, I understand. And I see, to my sorrow, that so many of my actions involved sacrificing my long-term values (for example, to spend time with my young family) to obtain what I perceived to be short-term success (such as producing a few more dollars of dental care, or attempting to please an unreasonable patient in the hope he or she would like me).

*Does any rational person wish for success instead of happiness?* Is such a condition even possible? Self-awareness can protect you from such errors.

While much remains to be said concerning the attainment of joy, I wish to begin illustrating my personal beliefs concerning the BUSINESS OF DENTISTRY. There are three essential ingredients, each of which must be mastered to obtain success in our profession:

## 1. Clinical Skills

You have already spent years developing these skills and have a career ahead of you in which to refine them. But even at this early point in your careers, be aware that **every patient who will enter your office believes you have the clinical ability necessary to treat them, or they wouldn't be there.** Certainly providing excellent dental care is essential to professional success, but patients who make appointments in your office assume you possess these talents, or they would never be seated in your dental chair. (They may indeed be wrong in this assumption, but they don't know that—yet!)

## 2. Behavioral Skills

It gains you nothing to be a skilled clinician and not be able to secure permission from patients to provide the care they require. Both you and the members of your team must excel in these "people skills" to obtain practice success. We'll discuss this topic at length as its understanding is ABSOLUTELY ESSENTIAL TO OBTAINING SUCCESS AND JOY. No dental care may be performed until a patient says "YES."

## 3. Business Skills

If you are the world's best clinician, and patients adore you, failure in dentistry will still occur if you aren't aware of the reality of our profession as a business. Do you wish to open a practice and be immediately swamped with patients? No problem—offer to provide care for them at no charge. But, you see, it is a business, and little dental care is forthcoming from a bankrupt office.

Often students are not only ignorant of the required business skills to run an office, but they seem to treat this vital information with disdain! This is a malady that must be quickly cured. Please allow the discussion that follows to begin your integration into the world of BUSINESSMEN, an honorable and essential calling.

What follows is merely a description of my personal philosophy. It is not THE best—not THE right one—but simply a snapshot of the beliefs I hold at this moment in time, after years of careful reflection. As I grow and continue to mature, my beliefs will change. Please read what follows with this bifurcated purpose:

1. To allow a better understanding of your author from a business perspective—my goals and beliefs.
2. As one possible philosophy—of an innumerable number of possible choices—that can lead to success and joy in our profession.

As we proceed with a discussion of financial freedom, using my office as a basis for analysis, let me make one thing perfectly clear. Many in our grand profession have created practices that produce and collect at levels which, when I become aware of them, seem unattainable—maybe even unimaginable—to a country boy like me.

But million-dollar production levels with 200 new patients per month have never been my goal. I'm a NET guy and I've maintained a simple and concise practice fiscal target for many years: to AVERAGE A NET OF $2,000 FOR EACH DAY I SEE PATIENTS IN MY OFFICE. (Just so we're crystal clear, net is what remains of total collected dollars when all the bills are paid, but before the pernicious effect of taxes.) This financial goal is one I have attained or surpassed for many years now.

Allow me to state that a maximum net in a minimum of time is not a goal to be prized by all in our profession. Some fortunate souls consider my work (dentistry) to be their recreation and leisure. They can't wait to get to the office. I find treating patients to be difficult, demanding and often frustrating. Many activities outside our profession are more enjoyable and rewarding for me. (Unfortunately no one will pay me much to do any of them.)

Other dentists wish to make a great fortune in the profession and will work 60 or more hours a week, sometimes 52 weeks a year, to achieve their objective. I wish them well. My desire here is to illustrate, not how to achieve financial success by continuous grinding effort (as attractive as that sounds!), but rather to speak for the attainment of maximum financial efficiency with a minimum investment of time and labor. If this clearly stated goal appeals to you, please read on.

Those of you who read my other books know I'm lazy. Recall that at the age of 40 I was free of all debt (including practice and home mortgage) and had over one million dollars in investments. I decided that was enough money to allow me to accomplish everything I wished to do for the rest of my years and reduced my time in the office to 80-90 days per year. (I heeded the sage advice that while money won't buy happiness, it will allow you to be miserable in some pretty interesting places, and among many other pursuits, my family and I have enjoyed extensive travel over the last several years.)

Since I'm often asked to clarify exactly when I do work, allow me to outline my schedule. I normally work three 6-hour days per week (Monday, Thursday and Friday). I don't cheat and work 20-hour days! That's sure not my style! I take every fourth week completely off, as well as almost all of July and August. I take off most of December, too, and every other day for which I can conjure up a reason. My point is that when all the dust clears, I see patients 80-some days a year and falling. (I anticipate enjoying patient care 60 days in 1996.)

Allow me to disclose the actual net figures from my office for the last two years. I think it only fair, if I choose to put my thoughts in writing, that the reader have concise and specific factual numbers to assess the accuracy and importance of what I say and not be left with a mere watery sketch of broadly stroked generalities.

I detest taxes and do everything that is legal to reduce what I must FORFEIT TO THE GOVERNMENT. Since my office has been incorporated for many years, I have a bit more leeway in reporting income than my non-incorporated brethren. I own the office space I practice in personally and rent to my corporation. I may increase or decrease the rent paid to me personally by my corporation and thus regulate the money that flows out of the corporation and into my pockets. We have a corporate year that ends on 30 June and this variation from my personal calendar tax year allows some opportunity to shift income. We take full advantage of both corporate retained earnings (a very complex, yet profitable subject to which I devoted an entire chapter in my first book, *Bringing Your Practice Into Focus*—hereafter *Focus*) and pension plans to reduce my personal taxable income.

The short version of the above confusing information for young dentists is that the income I report on my W-2 form is as low as I can possibly achieve, staying strictly within the IRS guidelines. Thus the W-2 numbers that follow are smaller than they would be if not for the IRS's zeal and efficiency at taking so much of my money. Even understated, the figures serve to accurately illustrate my point.

In 1992 my W-2 income from my practice only (not including any investment returns, retirement plan income or other sources outside my dental practice) was $174,000. I worked 90 days that year for a daily net average of $1,933. (Sure, I was $67 short of my goal, but the target was merely a nice round number I MADE UP anyway.)

In 1993 my W-2 income was $189,000. I worked 88 days that year for an average daily net of $2,147. (Author's note—this manuscript was written in 1994. It takes a long time to get a book from a writer's head to the reader's hands! My 1994 and 1995 W-2 income averaged $206,500 per year, on decreasingly fewer days worked, thus strengthening the validity of my point.)

As a result of my writings I spend a lot of time conversing with dentists on the phone. I am constantly asked why I still practice at all. Here are my "best guesses" in response to that often-asked query:

1. Eighty-some days per year isn't too unpleasant, even in a profession as demanding and exhausting (for me at least) as modern dentistry. Remember, my days are six hours long.
2. Who doesn't like money? Let's assume I sold my office for $400,000 and got cash up front for the full amount. I took that cash and invested it in a completely safe vehicle with a 10% return. My annual income from that investment would be $40,000. Now, even in this most rosy of scenarios I fall a tiny bit short of $189,000 per year. Yet I hear EXPERTS (who usually aren't practicing dentists) advising us to sell our offices and "get the equity out of your practice." In a clearer context this message could well read, "Sell the practice and pay me a commission. I need the money."
3. I started college in 1964, dental school in 1968. I've put a lot of blood, sweat and years into my profession. I am loath to walk away from such an "investment." Also, as I still practice I keep current. I doubt the many dentists/lecturers who no longer actually practice but merely talk about the profession can really keep fully informed, no matter how hard they try to fool themselves. Such superficial involvement is equivalent to the old advice of learning to invest in stocks by selecting specific equities, not really investing money but pretending you have and following your "results." Sounds like a safe and easy way to learn, but life simply doesn't work that way.
4. My wife of 25-plus years, Joann, can't stand me at home much more than I already am. She started working at our office when I cut back (mysterious coincidence), but she needs 80 days a year when she may safely stay home by herself.

The point of all the above foreplay was to set the stage for my explanation to you patient readers as to how I am able to net $2,000 per day in my small-town practice. First let me briefly clarify what DOESN'T lead me to this level of net.

I am no dental whiz! I don't do implants or ceramic inlays. Ten units of crown and bridge is a good month for me. I do the same boring stuff the great unwashed masses of you readers do—Pedo, Perio, Operative, plus a little Orthopedics and Orthodontics. My practice consists of bread-and-butter dental care, performed for middle-class families.

I am not suave, good-looking or a super-salesman. (Feel free to call my office for complete confirmation of this fact by ANY of my staff.) I bathe daily, try not to scratch when in the office and generally do the best I can.

Believe it or not, Keokuk, Iowa, is not really the Mecca of great dentistry—I just like to say that! I am one of seven dentists shoehorned in our little blue-collar village of 13,000. So what then are our secrets? I am glad you asked.

## A Productive and Profitable Hygiene Department

This is essential. I wrote an entire chapter explaining the concept of expanded hygiene in *Focus*. I understand that many of you are still in the position of first attracting patients and then searching for a hygienist. But the concept of expanded hygiene may be even more essential to beginning dentists. It will allow you to achieve more production from a part-time hygienist, while paying her a much higher salary—vital in the competitive venue of hiring these wonderful, but expensive auxiliaries—and reward you with a greater profit from her services.

We have two chairs devoted to nothing but hygiene and both rooms boast excellent physical facilities. We also employ a full-time assistant for my hygienist. I have had five hygienists grace my office over the years I've occupied it. All have been outstanding professionals. My behavior has been and remains problematical, but my hygienists have always been competent, professional and pleasant.

Our hygienist's pay is based on a percentage of her production. If she isn't treating a patient she isn't getting paid, so SHE has a problem. If you haven't ever paid a hygienist based on production, you will be amazed at their ability to fill open time when thus motivated. It's also pleasant to see your loyal hygienist enjoying a well-deserved cup of coffee and realize that, while you may have paid for the coffee, she isn't on salary while she sips it.

My hygiene department sees patients approximately 12 days a month (three days a week) and produces, on average, over $115 per hour. Thus I can count on hygiene to generate a minimum of $11,000 per month towards the roughly $25,000 that is our current average monthly office overhead.

## Associate Dentists

Again, my philosophy concerning group practice is covered in detail in *Focus*. I have had five associate dentists over a period of approximately 10 years and am totally committed to a group concept for many and varied reasons that we'll discuss as our time together continues.

The path of associate dentists in our office has not been as smooth as that of hygienists. Skills and temperament have varied greatly and there is the very real problem of doctor egos inherent in group settings. (My ego is certainly included.) My current associate, Dr. Lowell Long, has been with us for six years. He has been a real asset to our practice and is a fine gentleman—respected and cared for by staff and patients alike.

An associate is vital to my goal of $2,000 daily net as SOMEONE HAS TO BE IN THE OFFICE. Hygiene must be supervised, staff employed and patients cared for. My associate is hard-working, skilled and more than capable of filling my tiny shoes. I can rely on him to produce at minimum $20,000 per month, so before I even make one of my increasingly rarer "office guest appearances," our practice overhead is completely paid for, even in higher expense months. (For the math-adverse, or those just not paying attention, hygiene production averages about $11,000 per month, associate production is usually in excess of $20,000 and office overhead averages approximately $25,000 per month.)

The reasons one decides to accept an associate position are complex and unique to each individual and office situation. In our office, the advantages incumbent to the associate position include being immediately busy and productive from the first day. They have no need to deal with management of the office (administrivia, if I may steal a term from my good friend, Dr. Duane Schmidt), but can concentrate on the subject they prefer— patient care. They can show up, treat patients and accept a check every two weeks. Just like traveling with Greyhound, the associate can leave the "driving" to me. (We'll discuss the pros and cons of associateships at length later in the book.)

## Leadership

Now we get to the driver of our office "bus" . . . me. This is the venue where my years of experience are of most value. I realize that I run a business and PART OF THAT BUSINESS is helping patients to maintain a level of oral health they have chosen for themselves. For an office to be successful financially there are many concerns besides the mere treating of patients that must be dealt with effectively. Let's examine just a few of these critical areas.

### 1. Staff Meetings

Our office "leads the league" in meetings. It is through the staff meeting process that a true team develops. We have a brief staffing each morning before we begin treatment to review the care each patient is to receive and set the tone for our day. Our entire staff meets for two hours once a month. Our front office and hygiene teams each have their own additional and separate monthly meetings with me, immediately following the entire staff get-together. I meet with each staff member for an individual consultation several times a year to review their office accomplishments to date and co-develop a plan for their future growth.

While all team members are involved in these meetings, and everyone but the doctors takes turns leading them and taking notes, I accept total responsibility for the PRODUCTIVE OUTCOME of each session. These meetings require a lot of time and preparation, but they are THE essential ingredient that creates the synergistic energy which endows our office with continual growth. (Staff meetings will be covered fully in the chapters that follow.)

## 2. Office Monitors

We internally generate seven pages of office monitors a month. I don't believe a modern practice can be guided by "the doctor's instincts." When I go hunting in Canada, I like to take a compass along. I trust its guidance more than my "feelings" about the direction we must take to return safely to our camp. Our office compasses—the monitors—are compiled by loyal staff from the reams of computer data spewed forth each month, from our accountant's profit and loss statements, as well as from a number of other sources.

It takes my team a lot of hours to prepare these figures, but as the leader I need to be aware of possible trends in our office at a very early stage. We become alerted to any future problems by these hard, cold facts that compare current practice statistics to other comparable periods. Thus, we are able to intercept any unfavorable occurrences or continue to reinforce positive situations early in their development.

I spend a lot of time reviewing these numbers and all monitors are shared and discussed with every one of our team members during monthly staff meetings. The office belongs to all of us and our fates are mutually intertwined as regards its success or failure. I know in many offices all financial figures are deep dark secrets, reviewed by the doctor only late at night and behind double-locked doors. What if the staff discovered the office made a profit! Horrors!

I guess that means the owner-doctor doesn't trust the staff. **It certainly means they aren't a true team**, as I believe an authentic team may only develop in an atmosphere of complete honesty and trust.

What things do we monitor? Seven pages of legal pad size paper tells you we monitor a lot. Perhaps the best way to sum up the events we choose to observe would be to say we keep track of anything we feel could possibly be important to the well-being of our practice.

## 3. Personal and Continual Review of Office Expenses

I challenge every bill we receive. This discipline is obviously even more critical for a new dentist on a very tight budget. I don't order materials and equipment personally, but my staff know that while they may purchase anything they require to perform their jobs at the highest level of excellence, they are accountable to me for an explanation of why that particular object was needed and proof that the price paid was reasonable.

We'll discuss office overhead control in detail in a later chapter. For now, allow me to say that I believe **the opposite of cheap to be stupid**.

I gladly spend for that which is of value to me. Our practice is completely computerized with nine stations available within the office to input and access data. My corporation just purchased a Lexus for our president's (my) business use. I have made seven trips so far this year that include Greece and St. John for two weeks each, along with Charleston, S.C., and Scottsdale, Arizona. (As I write, my entire family is eagerly awaiting two weeks on a Caribbean Island with the intriguing name of St. Lucia.) The above listed investments of assets illustrate spending for things I value. Paying five cents more for gloves than we must drives me nuts!

## 4. Working Hard at the Business of Dentistry

I'm always talking to doctors who dislike the "business part" of dental practice. Please understand that in our current economic climate such feelings are no longer an option. Dentists, skilled and caring ones, go bankrupt today. Our D.M.D. or D.D.S. does not exempt us from such basic laws as supply and demand that govern the world of commerce. If attention to finance is too boring or beneath your dignity, I wish you well. Maybe you will be best served by finding a job as an associate of someone like me who will care for the business details for you.

The GOLDEN KEY to financial success is the realization that all of the above information can be summed up by this last scrap of advice: *See our profession as what it is—a business.* We must study business and devote a great deal of time and energy to this critical facet of being a successful professional.

Excellence in clinical care is essential to success in our chosen field, but in and of itself, it's no longer enough. If you attempt to be a dental ostrich, hiding your head in the sand and ignoring the business realities of a professional life, it's only a matter of time before something—most likely a lawyer or government employee—chomps on your butt.

To date we've shared my history, personal and professional philosophy. This groundwork done, let's turn our focus completely and intensely on the many dilemmas facing the beginning dental practitioner.

## Chapter Three

# To Solo or Not To Solo, That Is the Question

Enough of the philosophy and introductions. We'll certainly discuss the attainment of joy in many forms as we continue our journey, and there'll also be abundant opportunities for you to grow to understand me and what I believe. But now we need to focus on the first and perhaps most basic question facing anyone contemplating beginning a career in dentistry. That question which must be answered before all the others can even be asked is: Do I wish to go into practice alone or enter some form of dental group?

There is no one right answer to this poser. Both solo and group practices offer viable opportunities. But **there is one best answer for each individual,** and it's time to discover what choice is ideal for you.

As with all questions of great import, the key to divining the best answer lies in introspection—within the act of clarifying the values you hold most deeply. It will be upon the firm foundation of this certain self-knowledge that the best possible decision finally comes to rest, and we'll devote the chapter that follows this entirely to the essential, highly personal value clarification process.

Yet, some data must be gathered to facilitate arriving at your own best possible answer. The process of value clarification is a lifetime endeavor. Gathering the information needed to help you in this critical decision of which practice style best suits your unique temperament is the relatively quick and easy part. We'll proceed with that task posthaste.

Factors to consider personally when comparing a solo practice to a group include:

1. Do I possess an individual or group personality? Do I work well with AND UNDER others? Am I comfortable delegating tasks and performing as part of a team, or do I prefer to work on my own? What has been the dominant pattern in this regard that I have demonstrated to date in my life?
2. As the most junior member of a group, will I be able to submerge my ego to the will of the more senior staff? You may well be employed by a doctor who has invested decades of his life and hundreds of thousands of dollars building the practice you join. He will have selected and trained the staff and personally created every office policy. **The two of you will not be equivalent in authority.** Can you understand and accept this situation?

   Many can't and joining a group is not the best alternative for them. They reason they didn't go to school for years to be an employee. Yet these very folks may find themselves in a plural doctor setting some day, by starting a group practice themselves.

All individuals fit within one of four basic personality types. Entire books have been written on the subject, and understanding and identifying the various categories is critically important to allow dentists to relate optimally to every type of patient they treat, as well as enabling them to hire compatible staff members.

When you do further research on personality types, you will find differing names or titles given the four in various literature, but their essential characteristics will remain the same. It's important to be aware that no one category is superior to another—these are just the basic mind-sets with which we face the world. Each type contains its own strengths and weaknesses and is advantageous in some situations, a liability in others.

Let's briefly review these personality divisions with the immediate goal of identifying the most dominant trait in your own personality and then discovering the type of dentist with which you are most compatible and which would thus prove your ideal match in a group practice setting.

## Controllers-Directors

These are in-charge people. They are decisive, strong-willed, direct and controlling. They are focused on results and not too concerned about how their decisions are perceived by the people around them. They tend to be risk-takers and outcome-oriented. They are rather unemotional and may be perceived as insensitive.

## Analyzers-Engineers

Analyzers want all the facts and reach decisions slowly, carefully. They like to proceed methodically and become frustrated if rushed. They are unemotional, dislike taking risks and focus on details.

## Promoter-Cheerleader

These folks are fun-loving and care little for details. They are pleasant people to be around and keep both their spirits and those of the people around them elevated. They make quick, often emotionally based decisions, live for the moment, tend to be self-centered and are risk-takers.

## Supporter-Helper

Supporters don't want to make choices. They are greatly concerned with the feelings of others and are intensely uncomfortable with conflict. They are good workers and go along well with others' decisions, but become very anxious when forced to reach a conclusion personally.

No personality is totally within one category, but most of us have strong tendencies toward one division or another. Can you see that two controllers can't for long co-exist in the same office? Or how the supporter-helper would be most happy in an associate position where not forced to confront or make decisions?

Your first essential task is to accurately determine into which group your own most dominant characteristics place you. To gain additional feedback, you may wish to discuss with your family and friends the patterns your behavior has taken in the past. What is their perception of how well you have worked with others and how comfortable are you taking charge and making decisions?

Supporters are happier as group members, as they are relieved of the pressure of decision-making and confrontation.

Analyzers may also benefit from a group setting, as this allows them to concentrate on the details they so enjoy and removes the pressure of taking quick and decisive action.

It is difficult for me to imagine promoters surviving the gauntlet of eight years of college education. They are emotional people and lacking in long-term focus—but if they did survive the ordeal they would benefit from the stability of a group that would create a structure to help control their impulsive natures.

I believe the overwhelming majority of those who survive the rigors of dental school are controllers. These determined, self-directed individuals might benefit from a year or two in another person's practice—to enable them to learn the business of dentistry. But if the owner is also a controller, conflict between these two strong wills must inevitably occur. This factor alone may explain why dental group practices are so difficult to maintain successfully.

After you have assessed your own personality type, you must also develop an impression of the dominant traits of the practice owner you are considering joining. If the two of you are not compatible, there will be continuous strife and conflict that neither of you will be able to understand or eliminate.

While slightly off our immediate topic concerning selection of a practice venue, learning to determine quickly and accurately which personality each of your patients has is also essential if you desire to achieve success in private practice. With awareness and concentration, you will quickly become able to classify people into these basic groups. You must tailor the way you suggest needed treatment to patients based on your comprehension of their dominant personality profile.

The typical, even experienced, dentist explains care to each patient based on the *dentist's* personality type. This is logical as it is the way the dentist naturally perceives the information. But presenting all care in this manner affords a roughly one in four chance of communicating effectively. Not great odds when your success hangs in the balance. Let's briefly observe how acceptance of needed care can be enhanced by behavioral adeptness in this arena.

Controllers don't want to waste time! Give them a concise, accurate statement of their treatment needs; they'll reach a decision quickly and be ready to act. Too much talking just irritates these folks.

Analyzers want ALL THE FACTS. They may take days to reach a thoughtful decision and call back several times with questions. Be patient with these people if you want them to accept care.

Promoters want to know the BENEFITS of any proposed treatment. They are unconcerned with the facts—let alone the details—and will decide on a course of action quickly, almost randomly. They want to know if the proposed care will make them look and feel better.

Supporters are stressed by the pressure of making decisions. Give them the information needed and then assist them to reach the best choice. "If I were you I would . . . ." They're grateful for this help.

You will also wish to make use of this invaluable behavioral skill in selecting staff. You will be most compatible with people who process information in a manner similar to your own. This information may also prove useful to you someday in the selection of your own associate.

There is no absolute concerning how long you must practice before bringing another dentist into your office. It is not unusual for a highly successful solo practice to add an associate less than two years after opening the office doors.

My first associate joined me part-time during my second year of practice. It was not a good experience for either of us, because I had not thought out my goals or plans for an associate. I was swamped with patients and needed help! That's as far as my thinking had evolved. (It's not that my values weren't *totally* clarified—I hadn't made the slightest effort to even take a peek at them!) The associate and I parted ways, still friends, after a few months. My next answer to the "business problem" that beset me was to not accept new patients for the next four years. What business person—still in retention of all mental faculties—slams the door in the face of new business? I can now see better options existed. But let's return to our theme of selecting the type of practice for which you are best suited.

3. How quick a learner am I? How strong is my ego—how resilient my self-confidence? Can I quickly and comfortably take decisive action based on my own decisions? There is so much to master in a solo start. Identifying a community, finding an office location and negotiating a lease, designing the office, selecting equipment and materials, hiring and training staff. And let's not even mention the thousands of little details—like what color lampshade goes with the reception-room carpet—that will drive you nuts.

   Is this mental concept of office creation exciting to you, or does it fill you with dread? Within this single factor may lie the answer of whether solo or group is best for you.

There are two principal motivations to enter a group practice:

1. You are a group person—for whatever reasons—and wish to remain in this setting for the length of your practice life.
2. You want to spend a year or two mastering the clinical and business realities of private practice and saving some money in a group practice as you evaluate options for an eventual practice of your own. You are also aware that banks are much more likely to grant loans to dentists with some practice experience.

Either motive is acceptable, but it's imperative that both the senior doctor and associate be completely candid as concerns their plans. I think it unethical for either to deliberately mislead the other party concerning their intentions for the proposed office arrangement—be they long- or short-term in nature.

Despite your best efforts to visualize your future, it is possible your outlook will change. You may have entered a group committed to their concept and philosophy long-term, only to discover you hate it. Or you may have determined to strike out on your own after a year or two in a group, but find you are very happy right where you are. These are honest growth experiences, not deliberate deceptions.

## Dental Group Practices

The topic of group practices today really covers the waterfront. This can mean two dentists working together in Keokuk, Iowa, or 50 or more dentists in a large urban clinic. Also, some of the large clinics today are not dentist-owned.

I have had no personal experience with large urban clinics, other than having visited and read about a few. I don't feel it honest or fair for me to pass along hearsay opinions to you dressed up as fact. If a large group interests you, searching outside this book for more information may be necessary.

I think an important lesson for every dentist to learn is that no one can possibly know it all, or be all things to all people. (Humility admittedly comes easier for me, as I have so much to be humble about.) Keep this in mind when treating patients.

There is no dishonor in admitting you don't know—especially when you don't! Throughout this book I will clearly label as such any information I pass along that is not based on my own personal experience.

But I do know a great deal about small groups and I'm sure most, if not all, of this information will be useful when considering a large practice. After all, you will be comparing the large-group opportunity against the prospects of a small-group or solo practice to identify the best possible situation for yourself.

We will soon discuss in detail the specifics that should be considered in the evaluation of any office as a possible opportunity for you. We will also devote an entire chapter to examining the pros and cons of group practice as I have personally experienced it over the years.

But much of this book will focus on the choice of beginning a SOLO PRACTICE. This admitted bias is for two reasons:

1. Beginning a solo practice requires the most help, for reasons we have already discussed to some extent and will expand on in the chapters that follow. Also, much of the information vital to solos will also be of interest and assistance to those who choose a group environment.
2. I'm probably hopelessly outdated and old-fashioned. (My 14-year-old daughter, Megan, tells me I just don't get the 1990's. I tell her she doesn't get the 1960's. We're probably both right!) But I believe the dream of the great majority of dentists is still to control their own practice fate. This is admittedly tougher to do today, but still very attainable, especially if you haven't mortgaged your future with debt and are intelligent enough to seek help (such as the humble book you are currently perusing) with this endeavor.

There are two major ways to enter solo practice: Begin from scratch or buy an existing practice. There are advantages and disadvantages to each avenue. (Why is nothing ever easy and straightforward?) Let's take a careful look.

## Starting a Practice on Your Own

You will recall that this is the path I chose, in the now distant 1970's. (No, there weren't dinosaurs and we did have electricity. Folks were still sectioning third molars with a chisel and mallet, though.)

I believe to successfully follow this path you must be or become a student—quick and EAGER—as there is so much you must learn. You must enjoy a challenge, because baby, you'll have them. You must have outstanding skills in dealing with people and an acute sense of business.

You all have the intellect needed to begin your practice, or you would never have made it through professional school. But are you a self-starter? Can you proceed on a lengthy, imposing task with minimal directions (except perhaps this book) and follow it to a successful conclusion? Are you comfortable in dealing with others in situations like bank loans and lease negotiations? (I don't think confrontation is ever pleasant, but can you do it?)

Do you have the understanding and tenacity to educate yourself concerning sound principles of dental business? Because, unless there has been a sea change in attitude since my student days, you'd better consider whatever you were taught of business in dental school as merely an amusing interlude. If you won't force yourself to learn the business of dentistry (and I'm going to help you) and choose to begin your own practice, YOU WILL MOST LIKELY FAIL!

You must select a community, decide on a practice location and secure a lease, design your own office, select equipment and supplies, hire and train a staff—and thousands of minute details cascading on top of these. And, by the way, support yourself and your family as you are learning.

Each of the above tasks is daunting. It requires a self-confident person who sees setbacks, even failure, as just part of the learning process. How does one become this person? By creating a clear vision of your desired destiny and then having the courage to pursue that dream in the face of all the slings and arrows of outrageous fortune. It is the vision that provides the power.

Why would anyone, faced with the obstacles we've just briefly mentioned, choose to undertake such a task? (Assuming adequate mental health.)

### 1. You get to build the practice of your vision from the ground up.

Recall we've identified this as a watershed point. The concept of creating an office may thrill you! If so, and you have what it takes to get the job done, I personally feel this is, in the long run, your opportunity for the greatest possible success. (And by success I mean the attainment of both happiness and financial gain.)

Others may be horrified at the thought of all the *DECISIONS* that will be required. **Solo private practice is about a career of making decisions,** and often they will prove difficult (no clear right answer) and/or unpopular (all members of your team want one thing, and you—as head of the business—have to say no).

The ability to succeed on this solo path isn't based on dental class rank. I believe class standing has almost no relationship to private practice success. (However, this belief might be subconsciously influenced by my own class ranking!) They don't offer a grade for people skills and business sense in dental school. Of course, you must be a good clinician, but with applied honest effort and study I believe virtually every dental school graduate can become a clinically acceptable dentist.

Communicating and relating well with others, plus the analytical mind-set and strong will needed to steer a business to profit, are the essential prerequisites for financial success in any profession. Neither attribute played any part in the dental school process.

Pardon my redundancy, but *the biggest advantage in starting on your own is that you are the boss and will make every critical decision on the pathway to the practice of your dreams.* Again, does this thought fill you with excitement or foreboding?

## 2. It may be less expensive to start your own practice than to purchase one.

If you purchase a practice—a successful one—you'll buy all the equipment, supplies, etc. But you'll also usually pay substantially for "goodwill" in purchasing a thriving existing office. Goodwill is the purchase of patients, the office name and good reputation, etc.

No goodwill exists—yet—when you begin from scratch. How much you spend on equipment, new or used, is a factor you can control. If you choose to spend moderately, the expense should be less than purchasing an existing office.

## 3. Create your team.

We'll devote two entire chapters to hiring and then creating an office team. **Nothing is more central to the success of any office than the staff.** If you buy a practice you'll inherit the staff. They will be skilled and know the office, existing procedures and patients.

They will also, as normal humans, be committed to existing policies and resist all change. You may be able, given time and force of will, to get them to accept your personal philosophy of dental practice. But you'll sure as hell know you've been in a fight.

In the rural area where I practice, there are seldom any previously trained or schooled dental staff members that apply for jobs. I hire the PERSON I like best. If they have training, I'm thrilled! But I can teach them skills. I can't make them become friendly, outgoing, supportive. People either are that way or they aren't.

The staff you inherit will have been selected based on criteria developed by the office's previous owner. The coincidence that the previous dentist's values and yours closely coincide concerning staff selection is unlikely at best.

## 4. Your Philosophy

Maybe this is really a summary of all of the above. When you start with a blank page (or dirt floors in my own case), you can construct an office in your mind first, and then work to bring your vision to reality. This concept may have great, almost spiritual meaning to you. This freedom to create may indeed, consciously or subconsciously, have been what attracted you to our profession. You may already have a clear vision of the office of your dreams.

The idea may also leave you cold. Your concept of a dream office may be one where you don't have too many hassles and are fairly compensated for your efforts. All other concerns are just annoying details. I believe this is the line in the sand that separates solo from group mentality.

## Purchasing an Existing Office

A lot of the cogitation that goes into purchasing an existing office is similar to the thought processes of creating a solo concept, so we won't dwell on it in quite the detail, but let's take a pro-versus-con look at buying an office.

**— PRO —**

1. **INSTANT CASH FLOW.** You can probably very nearly end the list here. This is usually the main reason for purchasing an existing office—to obtain a steady stream of existing patients which means an established and instant flow of income from Day One. You can replace staff, equipment or remodel the office you buy and still eventually develop the office of your dreams. And as you are creating your vision, money is coming in.

   How long will you starve beginning from scratch? How much immediate cash flow will there be when you purchase an existing office? Determining the answer to these questions is where art comes into play. If you are painstakingly diligent in creating an office to begin on your own, and follow the advice we'll discuss, your cash flow can be almost immediate. Likewise, if you buy a successful office at a good price, you can be saving money your first year in practice.

2. **EXISTING STAFF AND DOCTOR THERE TO HELP YOU.** The doctor whose office you have purchased may stay for up to a year to assist you in the clinical and business areas and to introduce you to the patients. The existing staff will know how to run the office and also have a relationship with the patients. These items are part of the goodwill you paid for when you purchased the office and indeed are valuable assets.

3. **ALL OF THE OFFICE POLICIES, EQUIPMENT AND MATERIALS ARE IN PLACE AND FUNCTIONING.** About a million decisions are saved by these existing structures, and yet you remain free to make changes in any of them as you grow in the practice.

## — CON —

1. As we've discussed, the biggest obstacle may be if you can accept the staff you inherit. Are they your kind of people, with similar values and personality types? Will they be loyal to you? Are they willing to make changes to accommodate their new boss? There is often real conflict here, and it's no one's fault. The existing staff have a system that works and they're comfortable with it. Who are you—some wet-behind-the-ears baby dentist—to tell them to change? (Answer: The person now signing their paychecks.)

2. When purchasing an existing office, you undoubtedly won't have the ideal equipment and materials you would have preferred. You can adjust. In the army I often had to search for what was available to perform a procedure and simply conform my technique to the reality of the situation. It's amazing what you can remove a tooth with, if you have no other options.

   You will have bought the existing equipment at a depreciated price, already installed and usually for a significantly reduced investment when compared to purchasing everything new.

Equipment can and must be replaced someday, so you will be able to make desired changes over time.

3. The office facility may not be to your liking. No two people's tastes are the same. Maybe a purple and green color scheme will sort of grow on you? You probably won't be able to expand the office physically, but modification may be possible to create the office of your dreams as cash becomes available. You must carefully evaluate before you purchase if the problems you detect are situations you will be able to change. A new color for the walls is quick and easy to accomplish. If the operatories are eight feet by four in dimensions, causing acute claustrophobia in all who enter, there may not be much you can do.

4. Higher debt is possible than when starting from scratch. This is due to the goodwill expenses we discussed.

5. Will the philosophy of the senior doctor be compatible with yours? Did the previous doctor have an extraction, partials and dentures practice? If so, that care is consistent with the values of the patients who chose to go there and the type of dentistry the staff accepts as quality dentistry. Will these same people choose endodontics, a post and crown to save a tooth, or will they demand an extraction and a tooth added to their partial?

   How will you react when faced with this conflict . . . for the five-hundredth time? Be sure to observe the x-rays of current patients as well as actual dental work being done to discover the philosophy of the office. It's a big world out there, and indeed there are a lot of ways to skin a cat—or fix a tooth.

One of the first offices I considered joining was busy inserting an upper denture on a patient the day I visited. None of the patient's fourteen remaining teeth needed to be removed. I left as soon as it was polite to do so, and at that early point in my career, I was truly horrified by what I'd seen!

Let me throw in a thought-provoker for you—at no extra charge. If you purchase a busy office of a doctor who provided less than optimal care, is that a burden or blessing? Answer: YES!

It's an **opportunity** because of all the needed care just waiting to be done. If every patient in the office has ten crowns, what's left to do? But, what if they all have ten pin amalgams?

It's a **risk** because the existing patients came to this office for a reason. They may have had a PREVIOUS DENTIST who recommended a crown. Then old Doc Smith fixed it for a fifth of what the other crook wanted. Are you the next previous dentist? Can you do four-pin, five-surface alloys? Or do you have the business and people skills to have patients accept the dentistry you believe in? I can't determine your answer to these questions for you, but you damn well better know.

All of the questions we've raised eventually relate back to knowing who you are. You must carefully attempt to answer all the queries we posed so far. To assist you with this task, let's take some time and consider the absolutely essential task of value clarification, before returning to the specifics of beginning a practice. By then you should have answered the critical question of whether joining a group, starting from scratch or buying an existing practice is best for you, or at least be clear on the advantages and disadvantages of each.

## Chapter Four

# Value Clarification

The majority of my readers are perched upon what will undoubtedly prove to be one of the highest peaks of their lifetime. This is a thrilling time, replete with great opportunity and real danger. The effects of decisions made during this pivotal period, whether they concern life or career choices, are greatly magnified. Sound judgments will return your investment many times over. Faulty judgments may require years from which to recover and rebuild.

You are in a time of your life that DEMANDS cautious, careful consideration. But how can we develop the confidence to act decisively on these critical, life-altering decisions—often when there is no way to clearly identify any one choice as "right"?

As we have alluded, the key to creating confidence in our decision process is to develop a deeper understanding of our own innermost beliefs . . . our values. In truth, the decisions which face us now—the type of practice and location we choose foremost at the moment—are critical. But all of life is nothing more than the sum of the choices we make. Value clarification plays a much more vital role in our existence than merely helping us to deal with the issues currently before us.

Will you seat a crown with less than an ideal margin on a patient and tooth that are technically difficult to treat, or try another impression? Will you alter the date you performed treatment to allow coverage by your patient's insurance? If you join a capitation plan, can you live with the reduction in both quality of materials and time you can devote to each procedure that will be necessary to enable you to earn a slight profit? Or do you take a drug to feel better, or have an affair when your significant relationship is troubled?

The answers to all of these questions, and thousands more, will determine the course your life takes and if you will be blessed by joy or writhe in pain. As we will see, a life of joy results when one lives in such a way that the choices made are consistent with personal beliefs. But how can you make these value-based choices unless you are clear exactly what your beliefs are on every issue? You arrive at this point of certitude through the process of value clarification.

One last preface. The process we are about to discuss is complex. We will not limit our discussion to the simple problems of practice type and location, but draw on various examples that are, or to you students soon will be, a part of every practicing dentist's existence.

Value clarification is simply the task of identifying what we truly believe in. Be warned—it is not the task of establishing what we have been **told** we should believe in, by our parents, friends or television. Nor is it the identification of what we **wished** we believed in. Assuredly, the process is difficult and never-ending, yet I know of no exercise which will return as large a dividend in terms of added joy and success in life for your efforts. The method I use to clarify my own values is three-fold:

## 1. A lot of time thinking.

It seems in our culture today that quiet thought is a dreaded thing, to be avoided at all costs by many. Do you tend to have the television or radio on when you're alone? What is it you wish to avoid in your own thoughts? Do you like to be around people, or "busy" all the time? From what force do you seek to flee?

Peace and solitude in a location that is your quiet place is what's needed to achieve a better understanding of yourself, and to find authentic solutions to life's troubles and mysteries. This environment conducive to thought can be the library, your own office when no one else is around, or a room at home where you will seldom be disturbed. I have a basement study that is my quiet place of sanctuary.

Obtain such a place for yourself, whatever the cost. The only other requirements for this exercise are a pen and paper to record your thoughts, and if you like, a hot cup of coffee. Think deeply and often about who you are, and what you believe. Set aside a regular time, at least 30 minutes for this task only, at least once a week. DO NOTHING ELSE during this special time! Your mind will wander. Such is the nature of minds. It's very tempting to reflect on topics more interesting and less threatening than self-discovery. My favorite alternate topic is to reflect on how messed up OTHER people are. This is indeed much more entertaining, but unfortunately will not allow us to grow as a person, or prove helpful to those you are reflecting upon. (At least the people with whom I've been compassionate enough to share my perceptions of the problems that exist in their lives have never returned to thank me for my thoughtful assistance. Now that I think about it, they often don't even return.)

With persistence, this task of quiet reflection will become easier. Just continue to redirect your ever-wandering mind to concerns that deal with you alone. The daydreaming and loss of focus on the desired topic will lessen as fear of examining your feelings and beliefs decreases. Productive ideas will soon fill your note pad, each thought a potentially precious gem in value. We are currently focused on the type and location of practice we seek, but be sure to jot down any idea that strikes you as possibly important. You will be amazed what your somewhat quieted mind will bring up for your inspection. The one difficulty I have NEVER had to confront is having no problems in my life to deal with.

## 2. Observe your own behavior.

As the day goes by, and most especially at day's end, as you drift off to sleep, review your behavior and your emotions of the last 24 hours. Bravely identify those events which caused you pain, as well as those that brought you joy. The secret to happiness is to do more of the activities that bring joy and to avoid those which cause pain and don't help you to grow. Simple, but not easy.

If you fail to notice and identify the joy and pain, it's impossible to systematically increase the joyful, while decreasing the painful. *Awareness* is the vital first step to meaningful change. Don't fall into the traps of "false joy." Taking drugs, overeating, cheating on your spouse—in time these transient pleasures will result in long-term pain. Concentrate on meaningful happiness.

You may find real joy in such mundane things as patience shown or a kind word given or received. You must develop the ability to see through the short-term and observe that which creates true, long-term pleasure.

For instance, do you hate every day when you are scheduled to remove a tooth? I do. I spent a lot of years removing a lot of teeth. I took courses and studied exodontia, thinking as my skills improved, so would my enjoyment, or at least my comfort with the procedures would increase. Despite my honest efforts, my feelings toward tooth removals stayed negative. I no longer remove teeth. Instead I concentrate on performing the procedures I enjoy. Maybe unpleasantness for you involves certain types of patients, perhaps the very old or very young. Is it molar endodontics that makes you cringe each time you see the procedure listed on the day's schedule? Maybe it's a member of your own staff that day after day diminishes your joy.

Identify the pain and move from it. Perhaps you can discover a way to create joy in the situation. (Maybe you can discuss your concerns with your staff member. Perhaps taking a course on endodontics could help.) If you can't find a way for this painful event to bring you joy, my advice is concise: Remove the offending situation from your life. A bumper sticker I saw in Colorado sums this philosophy up nicely: "Life is too short to dance with ugly people."

Would you live with a cancer because it paid you rent? Will you continue to CHOOSE to suffer pain to obtain money? Or is the cause of your suffering your own fear of change? Clarifying your values will help here. I doubt life without pain is a possibility. What I believe to be possible is to minimize pain and also to deliberately decide when you will choose to accept unpleasantness, because the painful episode is part of a process that will, once endured, lead you to personal growth.

Do you wish financial independence? Does debt or a lack of money cause you concern? **Identify** that which brings you wealth, and do more of it. **Identify** that which reduces wealth, and do less of that. When you choose to spend, be certain that the purchase is consistent with your values and not just the result of some transitory emotion. If you won't do these things, then your alternative is clear . . . learn to find joy in poverty. At least accept the fact that poverty is your choice, a product of your collective decision-making in this area of your life and not something forced on you by sinister outside powers.

You students may participate by visualizing clinical experiences working with teachers or in team situations during your schooling. Are you comfortable within these groups, or do you prefer solitude? In athletics do you favor team or individual sports? Would you rather spend your leisure time alone or always be with friends? Begin to observe your feelings and actions and discover who you really are.

## 3. Observe and modify your values by awareness of your feelings.

The behaviors of others that make you feel uncomfortable contain the seeds of great knowledge. Their actions which leave you upset illustrate the parts of yourself with which you are not yet at peace. Let's take one hypothetical example of behavior in others you dislike and see how you can grow from observing it.

Do you hate "cheap" people? Then come to grips with the frugal part of yourself, and try to understand why it distresses you. Has someone told you that to be cheap is bad? Has the image of yourself as a free spender conflicted with a dislike of waste? It's neither good nor bad to spend money. This action is simply a choice you make. *Our feelings tell us how consistent our choice of behavior is to what our true values really are.* It is painful to have no clear guidelines as to our personal philosophy concerning the use of money. One day you are a consumer, the next a saver, each action frustrating the other. As is always the case, *unclear values cause confusion and pain.*

Allow me another illustration. Are you distressed by displays of anger? Then you're uncomfortable with your own feelings of anger. No amount of self-control can eliminate your anger, only disguise it. Emotions are not bad or good, they simply are. Use these emotional windows of insight to study your own make-up. The feelings you reject are parts of yourself that you have yet to accept. You have condemned them as evil, based on what is undoubtedly incomplete knowledge, internalized at an early age.

Take these discomforting feelings out of the prison of unacceptable behavior you have consigned them to, and restore them once again to their status as an authentic segment of who you are. A part whose purpose and duty you understand and respect, even if you may not esteem it greatly. Without the use of these parts of your personality, *you are incomplete as a person.*

Another way to employ feelings to help us mature is to observe our own behavior more perceptively. What are the authentic emotions, both positive and negative, that certain situations create in you? Examine and identify your emotions carefully, as these feelings can guide you in the choice of behaviors that will be most efficacious for you to select in the future.

Are the feelings you have appropriate for the situation or do they reflect childhood memories that aren't an accurate representation of existing reality? Feelings that may have been useful, even important at age four, may no longer be helpful to us today. Only by carefully examining our behavioral choices and our emotions can decisions concerning the efficacy and correctness of our current emotional states be reached.

I have always been uncomfortable with confrontation. My tendency is to simply avoid it. I now realize that often conflict can be helpful in the growth process. As you'll see later, in our staff meetings we use communication exercises that deliberately expose conflicting feelings. I still don't enjoy strife, but I am comfortable enough to no longer feel a need to avoid it, and thus can choose to use conflict constructively for my personal growth.

Maybe as a child anger was an effective behavioral choice for you to employ in dealing with your parents, friends or siblings. Perhaps it gave you control and thus comfort in difficult situations.

Is it helpful for you today if you "blow up" at work? Does frequent staff turnover or loss of patients from your tantrums now indicate that you need to examine this behavior to see if it is still appropriate? There may be times, as in a racquetball game, where anger can be productive and create needed energy which can be constructively channeled. In the aforementioned office situations it may be inappropriate and counterproductive. You have the power to observe your behavior, access the results, and plan whatever changes you feel are indicated to achieve the outcomes you desire. **Such behavioral awareness is called MASTERY!**

It is not appropriate to feel shame, guilt or as a failure in life because you were less than perfect at any given moment. Shame is a feeling we experience when we perceive ourselves not as people who acted badly, but as BAD PEOPLE. It is a feeling of utter devastation and helplessness. I suspect such an emotion often precedes suicide.

Such overwhelming emotions cause pain, but without allowing us an opportunity for growth. If you suffer from similar feelings, they are probably reactions from very early in your life. Freeing yourself from these destructive, but traditional emotional responses will be very difficult, but it must be done if you wish to attain joy and peace in your life.

It can be helpful to feel bad about your behavior. Therein lie the seeds of positive change. It is neither helpful nor accurate to feel you are a bad person with no hope of change. A condition of hopeless shame never truly exists, but is simply an error in our perception.

The first necessary step, which will allow us to grow by using the information available from our own feelings, is to identify **exactly** what emotion you are feeling. It takes both time and real effort for most of us to clearly label fear, tension, or slight apprehension. With attention and practice you will soon be able to quickly identify what physical sensations in your body are related to which emotion. How does fear feel in your stomach? In your muscles? Imagine or remember a fearful situation vividly. Try to identify the physical manifestations of that state you were in by recreating it at this later time. Repeat the exercise with anger, frustration, and any other emotional responses you are aware of.

Next, examine the appropriateness of your feelings. Some unpleasant emotions are earned by behavior on your part that doesn't coincide with your values. The discomfort caused by acting in a way inconsistent with personal values can guide us to more appropriate behavior in the future, and thus make our life more productive and happy.

Said another way, when we behave badly, we need to feel bad. This discomfort, if we don't ignore it, is our guide and mentor that pushes us to re-examine the behavior that caused this pain, and leads us to create an improved plan of action for the next similar situation.

I have days when I seemed dogged by a feeling of uneasiness. Usually this unpleasantness is accompanied by fatigue. It's only with great effort that I can continue through the day. If I take a moment, I can usually identify a particular event that initiated the feelings.

Maybe I didn't take the time to really do my best. Perhaps I spoke sharply to a patient or staff member and now I'm subconsciously aware of my remorse. The error may be correctable. Simply saying "I'm sorry" can make several people feel instantly better. Even a clinical failure can be something to learn from. Perhaps I should have rescheduled to finish the endo, or even referred that particular patient. Sometimes I discover that I did all I could, and my negative feelings are unfair to me, and after careful consideration, should be dismissed.

Whatever the result, the time involved in this introspection is a few minutes at most. The result is a much more pleasant day for myself and all those around me. If I choose to not reflect, I get to carry these feelings—like a bag full of snakes—throughout the day and often home and even into my bed. Which choice seems best to you? A few moments of quiet reflection to consider your past behavior and grow, or taking these "snakes" to your bed?

We can also mature by identifying emotions, such as shame and guilt, that cause pain but do not promote personal growth. Look back on your life and attempt to understand the beginnings of such feelings. Decide if these feelings can be of use in making your behavior more consistent with your values, or would best be eliminated by a better understanding of their origins and a conscious effort to be aware of why these emotions exist, and how destructive they are.

As we've said, if painful feelings don't lead us to grow, we need to eliminate them. Usually this requires understanding why these feelings persist (there is always a reason), and also the awareness that the reasoning which created these excruciating feelings was flawed or is no longer valid. Freedom from shame and guilt releases tremendous energy that can now be used toward positive ends.

Anxiety, insomnia, headaches and many similar disorders can be eliminated when the cause of the problem is identified and understood. Sadly, our culture has a bias to the "easy answers" and tends to prefer alcohol, sleeping pills, tranquilizers or destructive behavior to honest understanding and growth. Ask yourself where you reside in this choice of behavioral approaches. Do you tend to courageously face painful situations and acknowledge them as potential areas of personal growth or do you hide in the world of drugs, avoidance, or the blaming of others? I like to say the choices are akin to taking a shower (understanding and growth), or spraying perfume over the stink (techniques that attempt to cover, but not correct the problem).

This is a dental book, but I know that you can't be a happy dentist and a miserable person. Unclear values doom you to both a personal and professional life of frustration, fear, and uncertainty. Personal value clarification must come before, or at least along with, your office value clarification. That said, let me give you an example of how value clarification changed the life of my office, me, and my staff. Please remember that personal clarification is much more essential to your success and happiness, even if office clarification may appear less threatening.

---

## Our Purpose

Our office exists to serve the people we have dedicated ourselves to—our patients. We will create an environment of honesty and professionalism, where the patient will feel comfortable, cared for, and welcome. Every patient will be aware of the quality of care they receive and the sincere care of the staff for them.

We pledge to be positive, supportive team members and to create a place where we are able to have fun while encouraging and supporting personal and professional growth.

---

This statement of our collective values is framed and hangs in **every room** of our office. It took our staff a year to create this document. The reason its value is so significant to us lies not in the statement itself, but in the *process that created it.* I have had visitors ask if they can copy our purpose and use it themselves.

Certainly they may, but they have missed the entire point. It is the PROCESS of creation, not the product, that is imperative.

We began the creation of this statement with each staff member individually listing what each believed to be the central beliefs that made our office what it was. We also asked them to list what office and personal values they could identify, and what behaviors we could eliminate to move us closer to what we wished our office to be. All of these ideas were committed to writing and then reviewed by one individual to eliminate duplication.

With this list in hand, we met several times as a group and carefully discussed each point. Many suggested ideas were abandoned as not authentic, at least to the majority. New factors were identified in these group discussions and further explored. In the course of this review, many office policies were immediately changed, as we realized they weren't consistent with the office value core we were clarifying.

At last we attempted to create one document. Each staff member wrote out a personal version of our office beliefs. All of these documents were considered and discussed. Finally, a version that we could all commit to was drafted as it appears above.

None of the steps we took were critical. **The discussion and not the document is the point.** EACH of us was helped by the candid dialogues with our teammates to more clearly identify what we felt our office stood for. Each of us grew in understanding of our jobs, our fellow workers and ourselves during the process. The value of the team grew exponentially as we identified common values and thus created a common purpose to which we all were committed.

Did we make more money as a result of creating this PURPOSE together? While this document was drafted many years ago, I'm sure we did. The truth is that positive change in our office is almost always rewarded by increased financial gain. Did we grow closer as a group? Did we grow in friendship and understanding of each other? Did we share joy in the process as well as some pain? What do you believe?

Some chose to leave our staff during this growth process. The exercise itself didn't drive them away, but undeniably identified to them that they were in the wrong place. They didn't leave in anger. They left to go to a place where group values were closer to what they perceived their own values to be. Their leaving removed a great deal of frustration and turmoil, both in the lives of the team members who left and in those of us who remained. Once our values had been so clearly identified, the hiring of new people with similar values and beliefs was much easier.

The staff that chose to leave are still our friends. Two people can hold very different values and still like and respect each other. We wrote excellent letters of recommendation for the departing staff members, commensurate with the benefit they had given us as employees. We kept them employed until they found other work. These were good people and it didn't take them long to find other jobs, especially with our staff's assistance and support.

Over the passing years, two of the staff members who chose to leave have returned to our office family as employees. They seem to have missed the very thing that had bothered them in our office previously—the openness, honesty, and deep sense of a team mission. When they returned, their values had become very close to our own stated beliefs. I would like to think that they grew, and returned as closer friends than when they left. I believe the development of an office purpose to be absolutely essential if you desire a practice that produces a lot of excellent dentistry, rewards each team member financially, and creates an environment of common purpose and mutual growth. Without a clear purpose you can attain some of the above listed achievements, but you can't reach them all. Development of such a document requires a group that will commit to a difficult, often frightening and time-consuming process. It cannot occur without a leader (that's YOU, doctor) who not only has a deep commitment to clarifying the office values, but has worked through the clarification process personally.

Let me give you the sad news straight: You can't be a want-to-be and achieve this goal of value clarification in your office. This is not a task you can delegate to your faithful receptionist and expect it to be done in two weeks. The difficult journey of value clarification must be underway in your life before attempting such a thing in your office, or your staff will quickly see you as a manipulative phony, trying to achieve that which hasn't been earned.

Hard words, but true. To have, YOU must become. A central message of this whole book is that you can achieve whatever in life you desire, but only by personally earning it. You must first become worthy of success and then attain it.

Such a philosophy takes all the fun out of blaming others for our shortcomings. "My staff would never want to undertake a task like this, they don't have the commitment and the understanding!" Maybe you're beginning to see what they truly lack: LEADERSHIP.

The road I'm describing is messy, inexact, and difficult. It has no end in this lifetime. The motivation to embark on it is an unwavering commitment to attain joy. Is your life full of joy now? Do you share common values with your spouse? With your children? If you do, then your staff can work to create this self-understanding and growth. Can you comprehend such an accomplishment to be possible with all of the people in your life you care enough for to make the effort?

A world where you know exactly what you desire from every situation. A world where you are surrounded at every turn by people who know what you believe in and share many of the same values. Think of the joy! Conflict over values (such as do we stay late to see emergency patients, and do it cheerfully; or do we all arrive on time for work and in an ideal physical and mental condition, each and every day) has been eliminated by understanding. The energy tied up in these conflicts is now ours to spend on pleasure and growth.

Put away a tendency to argue, defend yourself, and win. These needs come from your apprehensions. Instead, confront your fear and use it to grow. Look deeply into your life and clearly see what has meaning to you. Help those dear to you to do the same, in love and not judgment. "Do the thing and have the power." Dare to create a world as you truly wish it to be.

I know these ideas are challenging to grasp, undoubtedly more so for those of you with less clinical or life experience. But value clarification is not a task to be mastered or completed. It is a process that will help guide you through the treacherous waters that are life.

These concepts will become more clear as we continue our journey through the book. Please keep your awareness of personal values foremost in your mind as we proceed. This is the secret to making the correct decisions with your practice and your life. Self-awareness is an essential piece of the puzzle that, when completed, reveals a life filled with joy.

## Chapter Five

# Our Town

I hope you've taken the time to carefully reflect on your values. I can well understand the temptation to rush through to the end of our story, as that's just the kind of thing I'd be tempted to do. I like to get things done. (A typical controlling personality—right?) But we are not involved in a finite project here, with a clearly defined endpoint. Instead we are engaging in a process. And as in the construction of a house, a proper sequence of events is essential. You can't add a foundation to your home at some later date, and skipping important steps of this process we're pursuing will rob the journey of its meaning, validity and ultimate chance of complete success.

So if you didn't take the time to start your value clarification, close the book and begin to make the investment—DO IT NOW. As we discussed, this is a lifetime exercise, but these quiet hours of reflection truly are like mining a vein of pure gold—an experience much too valuable for us to forfeit. For our current purposes, the only particular topic you must have clarified is the type of practice you prefer—solo or group. While it's never too late to change your decision, I hope you've dedicated some real time and effort to carefully examining your thoughts, at least about this subject that is currently so critical to your immediate future.

If you remain uncertain as to the type of practice opportunity on which you'll focus most of your attention, I'd advise you and your spouse—if appropriate—to go to a quiet place alone and STAY THERE UNTIL YOU ARE COMFORTABLE THAT YOU'VE REACHED A DECISION. ***Being able to make decisions and commit to them are essential attributes of all who achieve success.***

Fear of making a wrong choice paralyzes many into indecision. But, do you see that not acting is a decision too? As vital a characteristic as an action bias is the ability to continue to monitor and adjust your choices as the flow of your life dictates, so don't be rendered indecisive by fear that a judgment, once reached in this manner, can never be changed.

## Location

No matter what TYPE of practice opportunity you are pursuing, you must live somewhere. And geographic location is the next nut we have to crack.

In 1972, when I passed my Iowa board examination, I was licensed to practice in any state . . . as long as it was Iowa! The expansion of the boards into regions in years since has greatly broadened your selection of states available to consider practicing in without additional examination requirements. (Don't get me started on the stupidity of state and even regional boards. It does no good for me to bitch about this affront to our professionalism and only further elevates my blood pressure.)

With all these potential choices available, how are you to decide where to settle and begin to build toward your dreams? There are multiple factors to be considered, and again your personal values must be called upon to assign an appropriate weight to each of them.

# Geographic Factors

## Demographics

Demography is the study of vital statistics. For our purposes we wish to discover pertinent data about possible practice locations to allow us to make some key decisions, from the comfort of your own living room, concerning where we will consider practicing.

The best source of such data for dentists looking for an ideal practice location is the ADA Survey Center. You may reach this INVALUABLE RESOURCE by calling 312-440-2568. They will send you a free publication list that details all of the many surveys they make available. Allow me to briefly describe the three I feel will be of most value to you at this juncture in your profession.

*Facts About States for the Dentist Seeking a Location*

Does this title sound perfect or what? This survey contains over 100 pages of information including trends in population growth, taxes by states, dental license information and a whole lot more. The cost is $10 for ADA members and $20 for non-members.

*Distribution of Dentists by Region and State*

This data is also available for specific regions or county demographics, when you have appropriately narrowed your search area. Information contained within includes age and gender of dentists in each region, as well as number of dentists per area and what specialties they practice. The fee for this information is $25 to ADA members and $50 to non-members.

*Survey of Dental Practice*

This is an annually conducted ADA survey and contains such data as average income and age of dentists by region, type of practice, employment statistics and staffing patterns. (You might consider an office with seven staff considerably different, from a potential competition standpoint, than one with no staff.) The investment for this survey is $25 to ADA members and $50 to non-members.

Other sources of important demographic data include county planning and zoning departments and the most recent census tract information. Such statistics will allow you to see the growth rate in population of specific areas, average income and age of each resident and other essential information.

I would strongly suggest you carefully and consistently compile this data in your own market feasibility study. Any business considering a possible new location—every McDonald's or Wal-Mart—does exhaustive preliminary research before risking their money. Bankers will be very favorably impressed by this data and your businesslike approach as well.

You can easily compile data showing a pattern of above-average population growth within the area where you wish to practice. You may also point out an unusually high average income per resident and a lower-than-average dentist per population ratio, and that the area's existing dentists are above average in age. Sounds pretty impressive, doesn't it? And it will to a banker too.

## Family

This well might be THE FACTOR for some of you. A critical decision which must be reached is do you wish to live near your parents? I'm clearly biased here. Family is very important to me. My parents, four siblings and our respective families get together often. If you feel the same, I'd strongly suggest you stay within a maximum of 200 miles of your loved ones—close enough to drive there for the weekend.

If this is the case, take a regional map and draw a 200-mile circle with your home town as the epicenter. For what areas inside this circle do you currently hold a license? Are there areas outside your existing license you wish to consider, and are these currently unlicensed locations worth the #@$&^% of taking another board exam?

Some people wish to live near their families, but not too close. They want to be available, yet be certain of retaining their autonomy with the help of some geographic barrier. Such a concern by any member of your family also needs to be made clear.

## Climate

If nearness to family isn't an overriding concern, climate may be the decisive factor. Think in terms of the activities you enjoy—those that give your life passion. You can bowl or play basketball almost anywhere, but what about hunting, golf, tennis? Are there activities you really love where your opportunity to participate is defined by region?

Do you hate the cold winters, or love the mountains or seaside? What do you value? You can move later, but for a professional starting over, the time and money cost of relocation can be measured in terms of YEARS to recapture. Making the right choice the first time is imperative.

## Size of Community

I'm a small-town hick! NOTHING could get Jo and me to move to a city. "They're a great place to visit but I sure wouldn't want to live there!" I'm just as sure some city person would shrivel up and die from lack of neuronal stimulation in Keokuk. (No sounds of gunfire or high levels of carbon monoxide to keep the old adrenal glands going.)

No matter what particular portion of this grand land you choose to grace with your presence, the size of community you are most comfortable with is an essential consideration. Perhaps more than any other variable, population concentration will dictate your choice of activities—as concerns both potential area advantages and disadvantages.

We'll get to the professional opportunities of various sized communities in a moment, but think now in terms of personal and lifestyle preference.

Jo and I—the country mice—don't lock our home at night or even when we're gone for a few hours. We just don't bother. How important is that feeling of safety to you? (Who said, "Maybe you have nothing worth stealing"?)

If you have, or plan to have children, what about schools? Do you feel a large school with a plethora of available activities would be best for your kiddies? Or do you prefer the relative quiet and friendliness of a smaller educational system?

Do you like nightclubs, live theater, opera? Are professional sports your passion? All of these activities will be much more conveniently available in an urban location.

A small town offers quiet parks, relatively safe streets and a family atmosphere. I believe it's a great place to raise a family, but I'd have real reservations about moving to a small community if I were still a "swinging single."

## Professional Considerations

Let's consider small town versus city on a professional risk versus reward basis.

Small towns, if carefully selected, should give your practice a quicker start. Some significant overhead items—especially rent and salaries of chairside and receptions—should be much lower. But so will the reimbursement rates allowed by dental insurance companies. (A fact which is totally unfair, but nevertheless true. The same procedure performed on a patient covered with identical insurance is compensated at a significantly higher level in Iowa City, Iowa, just 95 miles to Keokuk's north.)

Cities offer much easier access to continuing education programs. Trained and skilled staff, especially hygienists and potential dentist associates, will be much more available, and often for a significantly reduced salary compared to what we small-town folks must pay for their unique talents. If your dream is to run a large office with multiple staff, population is a critical factor to consider. The chances of creating a five-doctor office in a town of 10,000 are slight.

Also, I read of marketing ideas and other practice-building promotions that sound neat, but are not something you do in a community where the other dentists are your friends. (I'm not about to mail practice brochures to an entire zip code that will include hundreds of my dentist-friends' existing patients.)

## Economic Factors

The cost of living, and of practicing, should be less in a small community. Rent and taxes—both on home and office—are two very significant expenses that will usually be greatly reduced in the smaller town. But fewer services and amenities are available. For example, the nearest dental supply company is a two-hour drive from our office, and when your compressor goes down, or some other critical piece of equipment fails, this is a major concern.

Also in a small town the personal wealth of the inhabitants will likely tend to be less. The percentage of small-town folks with dental insurance is probably also lower on average than in urban areas where larger companies are likely to offer expanded benefits.

But, again if you select the community wisely, in a smaller town you'll face less competition from other dentists and much less pressure from the growing nemesis of third-party payment plans: the HMO, PPO and other alphabet soups that are eating up an ever increasing percentage of dental services annually and seem to be the singularly darkest cloud on dentistry's horizon.

Allow me a sidebar for a moment. Nobody wants to participate in any of these initialed abominations. What makes them "work" is paying the dentist less for the same services performed. Dentists join these plans out of naivete (nice word for *dumb*) or from a desperation to get patients. **No thinking practitioner prefers these plans' patients to private pay clients!**

Keep this fact in mind when you consider these plans. Few decisions that are made in desperation, such as joining one of these programs in an attempt to get busier without the work of practice development, turn out well. Only the most efficient and skilled of businessmen have a chance of financial success with these plans, and these gifted folks shouldn't need to join them.

I recently spent one year treating patients from one of these plans. The plan our office joined had the highest fees of any I'd seen before or since. We tightly controlled the experience and kept careful records. I bunched all the plan patients together and saw them during one four-hour weekly period only. If they couldn't come to our office on Wednesday morning, they couldn't come at all. This restriction certainly didn't make the program members happy, but was an intricate part of my concept of being able to accurately gauge the financial effects of the plan before I ever signed on.

After a full year in the plan, our careful analysis showed that I had JUST MANAGED TO MAKE MY EXPENSE while treating these patients. In other words, working as effectively as I could, I was able to pay my overhead, but make **no profit**.

If you enjoy dentistry enough to perform it for free, that's great. These plans are for you. But let me warn you, I'm an experienced doctor and personally produce dental care at an approximately $350 per hour level (without including hygiene or associate production). If you can't produce at this level, you're probably going to be PAYING THESE PLANS FOR THE PRIVILEGE OF TREATING THEIR PATIENTS FROM YOUR OWN WALLET. Do you understand?

Now, after carefully considering the factors we've been discussing, and undoubtedly some additional items you've identified as uniquely important to you, a fairly complete and accurate GENERIC DESCRIPTION of the future location of your home and office should be developing. You've identified the basic area to consider (as near your family, or perhaps by an ocean, mountain or dynamite golf courses). You've also carefully considered the size of the community you prefer to spend your life in and have a clear idea if you are more attracted to solo or group practice opportunities. It's time to get out a map and begin to identify actual possible locations.

For example, if you're looking for a Midwestern city within 200 miles of your parents' home, you may find only one city to match that description. If you decide on a community of over

10,000 but less than 50,000 population, you may have ten possible sites to further examine. The potential locations will vary based on the selection criteria you've established, but at this stage of our process you have a manageable list of possibilities. What remains is the essential task of narrowing this field down to a list of final selections.

## Cover Letter and Curriculum Vitae (CV)

Let's get an essential fact crystal clear. Dentistry is a business, and any business lives or dies on sales. As a student, or recent student, you may not as yet fully comprehend this ESSENTIAL FACT. Or you may feel superior to this tawdry mercenary mentality. Perhaps you'll go into the world of academics where the state issues your paycheck. But if the dental clinic doesn't produce enough revenue—by selling its services—the hallowed walls of academia will come tumbling down.

Why this bit of moralism now? Because you are, at this precise moment, poised to enter the world of sales. The product being marketed is YOU. The challenge is to convince a dentist to bring you into his or her office and give you an opportunity. Or if you are starting an office from scratch, you must sell someone on the concept that you will be a good investment risk for a loan.

We begin the selling process with a CV that has one sole mission: To convince the reader of this missive that we are worthy of whatever consideration we are asking of them. This same information will also be important for our bank loan application.

Go to the library and research CVs. There are many examples available to help guide you as to the basic form of this document, but you need someone to BUY YOURS. It must be in some way superior to all the examples listed in the reference books. Let's see how this is possible.

You begin by listing your name, current address and phone number, followed by your educational accomplishments, listing the most current one first (i.e., go from dental school back to high school). List every academic honor you've acquired, no matter how tenuous its achievement, throughout your educational career. (I'd skip middle school safety patrol unless you really have nothing else going!)

Now list every employment position you ever attained. Pay particular emphasis to any dental-related experience outside of the required school clinic. I'm personally impressed by resumes of people who have worked and would strongly suggest you leave no work experience unnoted. The ten or so jobs I had before becoming a dentist did make me well-rounded and help me relate to people of almost any occupation—a significant plus. Be sure to list papers published or courses taken outside school requirements. (Perhaps you went to the Chicago Midwinter or attended a continuing education course offered by the college.) In short, note any event that may distinguish you from the madding crowd.

Next list any honors and awards not already noted, including captain of the high school eleven or debate team. Offices held, such as class president, really make you stand out, as they illustrate the respect of your peers and your own willingness to be a leader.

I would personally suggest you list activities, memberships and interests, including any charitable work in which you've been involved. Again, any signs of leadership are real positives. The world has no shortage of followers (or complainers for that matter), but leaders are always in demand. This also adds a personal touch that enables the reader (the buyer) to relate to you. (For example, I might note that an applicant likes to hunt and move her to the forefront of my list based on that dumb reason alone. That's how people's minds "work." We are more comfortable with people we can identify as being like ourselves.)

Follow this with a listing of PROFESSIONAL REFERENCES (not your mother) complete with their addresses and phone numbers, to make contacting them easier. The more impressive the listing, the better, but ALWAYS ask permission before listing someone as a reference and be certain they will give you a positive recommendation. A negative response from this list of people you have selected could very well eliminate you from consideration, and you don't want to work for anyone stupid enough to not check references. (We'll discuss reference checking at length when we get to staff hiring.)

The cover letter that accompanies the CV is a chance for you to describe who you are and of what your future desires and goals in life consist. DREAM LARGE! I would never be so foolish as to put down a single false statement on either the cover letter or CV, but think of them as Christmas letters—not an even-handed reporting of events—but a totally one-sided effort to look the best it is possible for us to appear without sacrificing our veracity. (The above sentence does much to clarify the concept of selling.)

Do you wish to serve mankind? Are you hard-working, a self-starter, dedicated, dependable, determined, etc.? Then tell your audience about it. Did you work your way through school? Brag! Do you have a special love of children or oral surgery? Maybe you're a skilled artist or musical performer. These things should be noted.

Now the entire package should be printed in **perfect copy**—NO TYPOS—and reproduced professionally on a top-quality paper. I'd suggest something other than standard white or tan paper, but nothing too wild. Perhaps an elegant blue. A few extra dollars and hours invested here could have an unmeasurable positive effect on your future. A nicely done professional photo attached to the CV also distinguishes you as a person and not just another application form.

Be clear on this: The CV won't get you a job, but it is what gives you an opportunity. The appearance of the documents should be clean and brief, with the words carefully chosen. This is a good experience in the discipline of doing things the best possible way. If you were the potential employer, and the person applying for your attention hasn't cared enough to create perfection here, why would you be foolish enough to consider them? If I'm an achiever and winner myself, I wouldn't. With our pristine CV now prepared, we can begin to narrow our search. The following is a list of resources to contact to help you locate potential practice opportunities:

1. Contact all the area dental schools near the region you have chosen. Ask for a listing of practice opportunities. Some schools make a real effort to help students and update the list of practice opportunities available frequently. Many just throw what they receive into a file that is available to you. The fact that you've paid four years of tuition to an institution doesn't in any way guarantee they will make an effort to assist you in beginning your career. They may not feel this is part of their job.

   Let's reflect a moment. How hard is it for a school to keep these listings updated and available? Maybe at the cost of two hours a month of secretaries' time? Now, how meaningful a gesture to future alumni (they'll still be asking you for money five years after you're deceased) is this small effort? Then, how stupid does it make schools that don't bother?

2. State and local dental societies may have practice opportunities listed. The dental schools will be able to provide the phone numbers of these organizations for you.

3. There are many professional practice brokers or consultants who are paid by the owner-doctor for the service of finding an acceptable associate for their office. There are a few national firms as well as smaller, regional companies engaged in this endeavor.

   While these can be real sources of help, **I would caution you here!** It is so easy to let someone do the work for you, but as is always the case, when you default responsibility you will pay a price. If you allow these firms to do all the searching for you, only a portion of the possible practices will be considered—those where the doctor is willing to pay the broker thousands of dollars for such help. Also, don't lose track of the reality that the brokers are hired and recompensed by the senior dentist. That's not immoral, it's just the fact of the situation.

Most of these companies list their services every month in the want ads section of the *ADA Journal.*

4. Dental Supply Representatives. I believe this to be a tremendous resource that is largely overlooked. Representatives of supply companies visit every dental office in their assigned area about twice a month. They have an accurate idea of how each practice in their territory is doing. It is also consistent with their self-interests to aid a new doctor in any way they can, hoping to EARN gratitude and thus future business. They can identify practice opportunities that may have never been advertised, such as those where a dentist is close to retirement but has not as yet made a formal effort to sell the practice, or an office totally swamped with patients that may wish to consider adding an associate.

   It was through the assistance of a dental supplier that Jo and I discovered our Keokuk location. The representative spent an entire day driving us around the area, showing us practices, introducing us to dentists and even buying lunch and dinner. We spent an invaluable 12-hour day together discussing the business of dentistry with someone who had years of experience in the field.

5. Area dentists. You can telephone dentists in the sites you have identified as possible locations and visit with them about local economic conditions. You can also discover if they, or any of their fellow dentists, are looking for an associate or may be interested in selling their practice.

   **CAUTION**: Some dentists may be less than candid, for reasons of their own. One Keokuk dentist told us he felt we would never do well here. Recall that we were booked two weeks in advance before we opened the office.

6. Want ads in such publications as *The Journal of the American Dental Association*, state dental journals, *Dental Economics* and others will list associate positions and practices for sale.

Now compare the list of economically viable locations you have identified (this task could well take a month of real effort and substantially increase your phone bill) with communities you wish to consider living in. You will, it is hoped, find a few matches, and this is where you begin your search in earnest.

You can contact individual dentists in your target area by sending your beautiful CV and following this up with a personal call in about a week. I would suggest you attempt to call doctors at home. Most have no time during the business day to take a call, and if they do agree to speak with you during their office hours, may feel pressured and bothered. If I did contact doctors at work, I'd do no more than introduce myself, ask permission to call them at home and determine what time would be most convenient for them.

When you do reach the doctor at home, begin the conversation by thanking them for their time and explain who you are and the reason you've called. THIS IS SALES. You must be able to converse pleasantly and establish some rapport. Remember, the person you are speaking to is just a fellow dentist and most are truly kind and helpful souls.

Have a written series of questions carefully prepared to ask each doctor you contact, and once you feel some rapport has been established, proceed down the list and record their answers. We'll get to the specifics of the questions in a moment, but by asking the same questions of each person, you can better achieve an apple-to-apple comparison from your multiple phone calls. If your conversation ends with mutual interest on both parties' parts, the next step would be to contact the local chamber of commerce for information regarding the community and prepare to visit personally. Most chambers will send you more information than you ever wished to know about any town, but recall who pays the chamber (the community) and understand that this data has the same level of veracity as our "Christmas letter."

I believe it is best to have found several possible offices to consider before beginning your actual visits, so you will have an adequate basis of comparison. Jo and I had identified nine practice opportunities before we began our first two-week odyssey evaluating each. Once this list of potential practices is complete, it's time for the personal evaluation process to begin.

## Chapter Six

# Visiting the Dream

Let's back up a bit and discuss the list of questions you will ask every dentist you telephone about a possible practice opportunity, as we discussed in the previous chapter. I've delayed the details of the list until now to make it easier for you to see how the data from three varied but vital sources of information you will gather about each potential practice opportunity will be integrated. The triple sensory input we'll discuss in this chapter includes:

1. The recorded data from the series of questions you ask every dentist while conversing with them during the course of an initial phone interview. Some candidates will be eliminated from further consideration on the basis of these questions alone as just not an appropriate match with your now clarified objectives.
2. The impression you and your spouse get from visiting what may become your future home town and talking with members of that community, as well as reviewing information from such sources as the chamber of commerce and your local library search concerning this possible location.

3. The sensations and information you get from your visit with the doctor, staff and office itself, as well as answers to another precise set of questions prepared in advance specifically for the office visit which we'll detail in a moment.

If you are married, I strongly urge you to include your spouse in all of these essential fact-gathering missions. The decision you'll soon be making will have a tremendous impact on both your futures. Such pivotal choices must not be made unilaterally. Of course, two sets of senses will comprehend more than one, and while you are meeting with the doctor, your spouse may be finding out what is REALLY going on in the office from the best possible source—the staff members.

Another caution: You must make every effort to **SELL YOURSELF** to each office you evaluate. Until you have completed all of your visits, it's difficult to determine what your final choice of practice to join will be. If every office you visit offers a position, you find yourself in the lovely position of selecting from among the multiple offers tendered. That is a lot less painful situation than having every doctor turn you down.

It's tempting to dismiss an office that you feel may not measure up to another practice you've already visited, and thus not bother to thoroughly investigate this possibility and risk giving the dentist-owner the impression you would not consider the practice. But be very wary of such a mind-set unless you have a firm employment offer from another doctor.

So dress in an acceptable fashion to impress the (usually older) doctor who will have the final say as to your job prospects. This is not the time to make a fashion statement about your true inner self! Be friendly and outgoing. Show your appreciation and enthusiasm for what this office has accomplished. Avoid making any judgments or criticisms of the office, at least out loud, if for no better reason than the Golden Rule. In every encounter remember, this office has something you desire. You are the seller, they are the buyers. This is simply the reality of the situation.

Now on to the specific queries for our initial phone interview. Recall that we have chatted for a while—the longer the better—and established rapport before beginning any questions. Often the doctor will have already inquired about your own history and future plans. Because of the value clarification process you've been involved in, you should have some fairly definitive answers. ("I don't know," may be candid, but is hardly impressive!) Individuals with a clear, and thus dynamic, vision of their future can't help but be seen in a more positive light.

When you feel comfortable, proceed with your list of questions, but don't ask them pedantically, as a teacher giving an examination might. Shape these questions so they flow naturally into the conversation, but be certain to get the answers you need and *record the data.* Weeks later you won't be forced to rely on memory when you visit this office or try to recall which doctor told you what three weeks ago.

## Phone Questions for Possible Employer

### 1. Would you please tell me about your office?

All of the questions that follow will be of the *open-ended variety* (i.e., where yes or no answers aren't possible) to allow some freedom in response as well as to encourage the doctor to provide more information. This will give you a better opportunity to evaluate, not only the information you are receiving, but the person presenting it. The type of specific data you wish to obtain from this very broad query, and which you may need to ask additional follow-up questions to discover, includes:

a) How long has your office been located in this community? Length indicates stability, but a younger, fast-growing office is also definitely an attractive possibility. We'll discuss how to gauge practice growth in a moment based on data obtained during the office visit itself.

b) Is this the only office location in which you've practiced? If not, why was a move made? No doctor likes to relocate a practice. It's a massive headache and a total disruption of income. Frequent moves are a real red flag of caution that something is wrong. Of course, moving across town to a more rapidly growing area and a larger, nicer office is hardly a cause for concern.

c) Tell me about the size of your office facility and how is it equipped? You'll learn much more during your actual visit, but a BARE MINIMUM of four operatories and 1,000 square feet would be required for two dentists and a hygienist to coexist. Less available space than this might eliminate an office from consideration.

d) Do you have existing space for another dentist and is that area already fully equipped? Again, you'll have to examine the available equipment personally during your office visit to determine if it is suitable. It is hard to feel good about yourself personally, or impress the patients you treat, if the area you are assigned to work in is noticeably less attractive than the remainder of the office.

e) What special procedures in dentistry do you personally most enjoy?

f) Are there particular dental specialties that you would expect or wish me to take over?

From the answers to the above two questions, how do you feel you two mesh professionally? If Doctor Senior wants you to perform all the pedo and oral surgery, and these are two dental procedures you dislike, you have a limited future together! The same would hold true if you both enjoyed crown and bridge, and end up fighting for the same patients. The ideal is when the interests of both doctors complement each other.

## 2. What plans do you have for the future of the office?

With this question you wish to determine what the doctor's vision of the future may hold for YOU. Does he or she plan to retire in two years and wish to sell the office? Or is the practice still in a rapid growth phase with you being one of a number of eventual associates or perhaps partners? Either of these answers could be construed as good or bad, depending on your interests and perspective.

Obviously, if you want to be on your own soon, joining a 35-year-old dentist still very much into practice expansion is less than ideal. Likewise, if you don't wish to go on your own, or you feel you are too deeply in debt to consider buying into a practice, the doctor near retirement scenario will not be to your liking.

## 3. Have you employed previous associates?

In some ways it's nice NOT to be the initial associate dentist. There are many problems to be worked out the first time through an associate arrangement, both logistically and philosophically.

By logistics I mean adding equipment and staff. Also, existing staff must make adjustments to the extra pressure created by the presence of additional people—both staff and patients in the office—and further demands on their current jobs. They may well be asked to work evenings and Saturdays, and may not like it!

There are also less tangible but very real problems such as having an employment contract drawn up. Remember that the senior dentist may be as new to this associate thing as you are. Being able to do a crown preparation in 20 minutes doesn't mean you know the ideal way to introduce another doctor to your office!

I personally had no "voice from above" instructing me how to proceed with my first associate. It was strictly done by extreme trial and not a little error.

Philosophically a problem exists for the senior doctor as to how much supervision of the new dentist is appropriate. The patients the associate treats have usually come to the office expecting to be seen by the senior doctor, so the owner-doctor will have a personal as well as legal reason to be very concerned about the quality of care being performed. Too close a supervision sends the message to the associate, staff and patient that you don't trust the person you have hired. The need to check their work also adds a great deal of stress to both doctors' days. (Believe me, I know!) Providing just enough assistance without interfering is easier said than done.

The associate may be uncertain when to seek help or advice, without appearing incapable to patients, staff and employer. Let me give you a clear guideline for this problem: If the patient's care can possibly be improved by asking for assistance . . . ASK. To give the best care we are capable of is our imperative legal, ethical, moral and professional duty. If the senior doctor isn't glad to assist you, both for your sake and the well-being of your patients, you have made a poor choice of offices.

The senior dentist is also faced with the dilemma of how to entice the patients who have come to see him, to accept appointments with the new associate. This is not a simple task, and we will discuss the proper way to ensure this happening in detail later on, but it involves concerted effort by both doctors as well as other staff members. If this delicate issue is handled poorly, the ultimate result can be a significant number of patients leaving the office entirely.

From my own perspective as the senior dentist, there was a great deal of turmoil and heartache involved in bringing in my first associate. There were many times when I wondered if I'd made a terrible mistake.

If you are the first associate ever employed in an office, be aware of the difficulty and uncertainty the owner is dealing with. I once thought parents knew everything, until I became a struggling, laboring parent myself. It may be easier for you to understand the need for some adjustments to be made after you begin employment, having an awareness of the senior doctor's blind struggle to find a system that will be equitable for everyone involved.

Yet, while being first can be tough, you must be concerned if other associates have come and gone from the practice. Quality associate relationships are very difficult to maintain. While my current associate has been with us six years, he is the FIFTH associate I have employed. One critical question to ask a doctor who has had multiple associates come and leave, is how long did the former dentists stay? With one exception, all of the associates I employed stayed about a year and left to pursue independent practice opportunities and established offices of their own. I hope they learned a little in their time with us that helped them to be both more successful and happy.

All of the associates we have employed have been real assets to our office, with the sole exception of a young man I felt very confident in hiring, but the experience proved to be a disaster for both of us. We'll deal at length with staff hiring in a later chapter and you'll see that no matter how hard you try to establish an ideal match between people, it is much more an inexact art than a science.

If several associates have left after a few months in any office, I'd be very concerned that problems exist within this practice that have led to these early departures. You'll undoubtedly want to know why the previous associates left. Be aware that the senior doctor may not really know, and even if he does, may give you the now famous (to us) "Christmas letter" version of an answer. (By this I mean a response more notable for showing the office in the best possible light than for its candor!)

Ask permission to contact past associates. The office will have their addresses and phone numbers. Be aware that their answers to the questions you ask about the office and why they left will also be of the "Christmas letter" variety.

## 4. Existing staff

How many staff are currently employed? How long have they been there? What plans does the doctor have for staffing the new associate? NO DENTIST SHOULD EVER WORK WITHOUT A CHAIRSIDE, especially when beginning in practice. I refuse to allow even a sealant to be placed by my hygienist without assistance. My hygienist is very skilled, but there is no way the quality of the work she performs alone can consistently equal that done by her with the aid of a skilled assistant.

Also, I believe it vital that young practitioners have someone working with them for emotional support as they struggle valiantly with the very difficult job of modern dentistry.

Frequent staff turnover, just as associates leaving quickly, would constitute a red flag of warning that may indicate internal office troubles. If several staff have been employed less than a year, unless they are additions to the staff rather than replacements, I'd be wary. **No one should accept a job where they don't feel they can have fun! People don't accept positions to leave them, and frequent turnover is often a sign of an unpleasant working environment.**

## 5. What is the philosophy of dentistry your practice espouses?

Is the office oriented toward prevention or dentures? Do they fabricate more crowns or partials? How do they perceive the patients who trust them for their care? As honored guests or a stupid and inconvenient problem to be dealt with daily? (Many offices grow to the point where they view the patients as an annoyance, as foolish and self-destructive as that may sound.)

Of course, you're searching for a match between **your clarified personal and professional values** and the philosophy of the office. If your philosophy revolves around prevention, perio and crowns, and the office takes pride in the fine quality of the dentures they create, a smooth relationship is unlikely.

PERSONAL OPINION: I dislike to hear an associate inquire about a guaranteed salary, especially early in our discussions. Of course, as the relationship between the two doctors develops and substantial hope of reaching an agreement emerges, a firm contract that spells out salary and many other factors must be clearly established. But bringing compensation up too early in the discussion gives the appearance that income is the highest priority for the candidate. That is probably not true for most of us and usually will not be seen in a positive light by your potential employer. Also, asking for a salary guarantee indicates to me a lack of confidence by candidates in their own abilities.

Please understand, I have nothing against a guaranteed minimum salary. Even asking for a salary advance of a few thousand dollars is acceptable if personal financial needs so dictate. (Although it is imperative that concise arrangements for this debt's repayment from future office earnings be established, and that the loan be erased within a matter of months. Unpaid debt between doctors is an unneeded strain on this delicate relationship.) We'll discuss contracts and such specifics later. But giving the perception that income is more important than a quality work environment and the opportunity to care for patients is deadly to patient case acceptance and not the impression you wish the staff and doctor of a potential employment opportunity to develop.

It certainly is appropriate to ask senior doctors, as your conversation comes to an end, what their feelings about your suitability for the office may be at this early juncture. They may be unable or unwilling to divulge this information at this time, but there is also a chance you will receive a very candid answer that will prove helpful in your decision-making process, whether the response is positive or negative in tone.

As you hang up the phone, review and clarify your notes. Summarize them, and ask yourself this critical question: DO I LIKE THE PERSON I JUST FINISHED TALKING TO? Is this person one I feel a bond with and with whom I'd choose to spend a lot of future time? Were they candid and open in the discussion? Do I **trust them**? These right-brain impressions are as important to the final decision as any of the "facts" you have recorded in your notes.

## Visiting the Dream

You have located a good number of potential practice sites and contacted the owners by phone. Several were eliminated as not right for you, but most were deemed worthy of future consideration. Finally it is time to physically visit the community and office where you may begin your career. It should be an exciting moment!

As you prepare to visit your potential new home, I have two suggestions I feel are very important:

1. As I've repeatedly stressed, this is an assignment for you and your spouse. Whatever the difficulties—missing work, finding a sitter—surmount the obstacles and both of you be involved in every step of this journey.
2. Visit the office, at least for an hour or two, when the staff is present and patients are receiving treatment. This is the only situation you really need to evaluate, not how nice the office looks after the cleaning lady leaves. The **function** of this business is of much greater import than its form.

It is essential to gain a sense of the atmosphere of the practice while it is working. Trust your instincts, good or bad. That's exactly how patients decide if this is the office for them. Also, your liking the staff and their liking you is more critical to your future than it may be possible for you to understand at this juncture. Staff can, and will, make or break you.

If you become a dentist in this office, after you examine a patient, recommend some care, and then leave the room, the patient will ask the staff about you. Is she gentle? Is he good? Not just the words, but the inflection of the staff's answer can decide if that patient will accept you as their dentist. There are about 100 other ways staff will be instrumental in your future that I'm aware of, and undoubtedly 900 more I don't have a clue about.

Trust me! Getting along with staff is essential to your success. Be on your very best conduct for this first crucial impression. There is an understandable tendency—perhaps due to nerves or insecurity—to come off a little superior to the staff. To do so is the kiss of death. Never forget the staff of this office may become your co-workers and friends.

3. Allow at least an hour, better two, to examine the town in daylight. The information from the chamber of commerce and possibly the library should give you an idea of what specific sites you need to observe. This is the community in which you're considering spending your life. Certain physical necessities may be essential for you to attain joy. (This may seem a petty example, but I wouldn't personally consider living in a community without excellent tennis courts.)

What follows are my suggestions for information you should be clear on concerning the community, either from your research, asking local citizens, or visual inspection of the town itself. This list must be augmented by things you consider essential for your and your spouse's personal well-being. For me, "How's the hunting?" and "Let's see the tennis courts" would about do it, but I was brought up poor and remain an easy guy to please. I'm sure the quality of the country club would be as vital to many young doctors.

1. WHAT IS THE TREND OF THE LOCAL ECONOMY? A community growing in size sure helps any beginning business, and **you are about to become a new business, remember?** Are there current or recently past strikes or labor problems? Do you find new, especially large businesses opening facilities? Is there one dominant employer, that if closed would kill off the economy, or like Keokuk, are there multiple employers of moderate size? Hard times come to every business . . . ask the folks in Detroit. A one-business town is Heartbreak City when the one business is going bad.

2. Ask around town concerning the reputation of "ole Doc Smith." At least in a small town, everyone will know Doc. They'll tell you both good and bad. In our little town they can tell you which doctor takes a sip now and then or has a girl friend. What you'll hear—and ask everyone you meet, including the guy at the gas station, to get the broadest possible sampling—will soon tell you the reputation of the office you

are considering joining. If nobody around knows who Doc Smith is, wouldn't that worry you a bit?

3. Look the town over. Is it growing, with new areas of homes and industry being developed? Or do you see a lot of storefronts boarded up and a whole lot of for-sale signs in people's yards? (No matter what they tell you, there is NO indigenous shrub that resembles a for-sale sign!)

   You can become successful in a town that isn't growing, given hard work and time. But it's like swimming against the current—you have to work pretty hard just to hold your own. Why would anyone CHOOSE to enter a shrinking community or practice? No matter what percentage of production the doctor offers you as compensation, if there are no patients to care for, it's academic.

4. Pay special attention to the situations you've personally identified as important. It may be the schools, YMCA, tennis or golf facilities, country club . . . whatever your unique interests dictate. Don't hesitate to talk to school officials, ask about Y programs for all your family, or do whatever else is required to feel comfortable with the situation you are observing. **Making decisions that will deeply affect your family's future is not a time to be timid!**

Now you and your spouse ask each other, DO YOU LIKE THIS TOWN? Does it smell nice (not like a paper or grain mill)? Is it clean and neat? Do the people seem friendly? Did you see people on the streets who worry you?

There is a tendency to block out or minimize areas of possible trouble. Keep all four of your eyes open, and make your best honest judgment of the situation. I remember Jo and I didn't sleep much in one town we visited due to the roar of motorcycles past our hotel all night long. This kind of "data" is important! Do you wish to raise a family in a town where all-night motorcycle activity is a problem?

At last we pull up in front of Doc Smith's office. It's crunch time. Spend a minute and complete your notes about the community. Compare observations and opinions. Then begin to look ole Doc over right from your car. Does the office area have plenty of PARKING available? This can be essential, especially in some urban settings. A second doctor will only exacerbate an existing parking problem. Does the front of the building look pleasant and professional? Is the grass cut, and the lawn free of debris? Can you see the practice sign from the street? If not, that may need to be changed.

Of course, you are punctual or even a few minutes early. If you've never been on time in your life, be so now, even if it means leaving at 4 a.m. to get there promptly. I feel the best time to visit any office is mid-afternoon. This affords you the opportunity to see the office in action, and then let poor old Doc calm down after a busy day and converse with you in peace and tranquility. At the end of the day you'll both have as much time as needed to complete your discussion.

As you enter the building, continue to allow your observations to accumulate. Note the hallways and especially the door to the office. Note the sign on the office's door. What are your impressions?

Enter the office and look around. Is it busy? YOU SHOULD BE GREETED BY NAME FROM A STAFF MEMBER WITH A BIG SMILE ON THEIR FACE WITHIN A MINUTE OR TWO OF YOUR ARRIVAL.

If you aren't greeted warmly, and by name (assuming you're on time), this staff isn't going to do so for their patients. And virtually every successful office gets this critical step right. You want to let each patient know immediately you are glad to see them, and that you value them as individuals. No sound is sweeter to the ear than that of your own name!

Introduce yourself and your spouse to the receptionist and then let this capable staff member take over. The receptionist is the critical ambassador of the office and should be completely comfortable and in control in this situation. The doctor may have asked her to seat you in his or her private office until he or she has completed a procedure and has time to greet you personally. He or she may have advised her to show you around the office and introduce you to the rest of the team. Whatever the case, the receptionist should be firmly in charge and you both her gracious guests.

Some doctors prefer you not bother them or the patients they are treating. This wish must be respected. Your visit should in no way interfere with the function of the office. This is unfair to patients and won't endear you to the staff! Other doctors (myself included) aren't bothered at all if you wish to observe them at work. The gentleness, compassion and relationship between the doctor, staff and patient are the key points you wish to note, not if the old guy can place a class two alloy. Whatever the case, do as you are asked. Keep your senses alert and you will learn a great deal from any vantage point in a dental office. (Frequent screams—even by the doctor—would represent a clue of some significance!)

What follows is the last LIST of information you must gather to properly evaluate this business opportunity. This final data may be the most essential of all your input. You must make an effort to obtain all of these facts if you are in any way serious about joining the office. Again, be pleasant, but not timid. If the doctor says the facts you request aren't available, so be it. But the data we'll be talking about is information every successful office is aware of, and if the doctor is forthright, he or she will probably be glad to provide it for you.

The following information is listed in no particular sequence or priority. Your personal values must assign the appropriate weight to each variable. Some of the questions were previously asked during the phone interview, but in the office the doctor has direct access to the information, whereas on the phone he or she must rely on memory. Also, it's very interesting if the phone answers you recorded differ from the ones given to the same questions asked in the office.

1. Doctor, we've really enjoyed meeting your staff. They have been most gracious! Could you tell me a little about each one, what their function is in the office AND HOW LONG THEY HAVE BEEN WITH YOU? (We've already discussed the importance of staff longevity. You or your spouse can also ask the staff the identical questions. I would also ask each staff member if they feel this is a good place to work and if they are happy.)
2. Does the practice participate in any managed care plan? What percent of the office revenue would such plans make up? What involvement on my part do you anticipate with these particular patients?

   Remember, these are the programs that make it very hard to make a profit. If the answers to the posers above are that 50% of the total office is involved with plans, and we expect you to do 100% of that care, you're out of that office early! Be aware that bringing in another dentist to treat these unprofitable third-party patients is a common reason to seek an associate.
3. Could you give me some idea of the economic condition of the office? How much debt is being carried?

   Now, this is clearly none of your business, *unless you plan to join the office,* which happens to be why you are there! Many of you will be uncomfortable asking this, but it is the most basic of BUSINESS QUESTIONS, and not an invasion of privacy. If you are to move your family to this community and join the business, you have a right to know if the office is going to go broke!
4. Would you please refresh my memory about your previous associate experiences? How many, how long did they stay and why did they leave? We've discussed the significance of this information previously. You can expect a more detailed explanation in office, after there has been time to research the needed information, than was given off the cuff, over the phone.

5. What plans do you have for assigning me patients? How busy has the office been in the last year? Of course, these two questions are CRITICAL. We will ask to see the profit and loss statements in a moment, and they will clearly illustrate if the office is growing or declining and thus either verify or disprove what the doctor has told you. If no plan exists to get you patients (and if you are the first associate, there may well not be one), somebody better be working on a system. We'll give you very valuable advice on how this delicate task is best performed a bit later.

6. What are your personal future plans for the business? Again—retirement, bringing in more associates, or is adding one other dentist the end of the dream? Plans can change, but you deserve to know the current status of affairs that will profoundly affect your future.

7. THE CONTRACT. If one has already been drawn up by an attorney, you should be given a copy to review with your own lawyer. **Drafting a contract is not a do-it-yourself task for a dentist who thinks he or she should have been an attorney.** Neither is reviewing it on your own. I hate lawyers as much as any among you, but their services are essential here. (Much as it pains me to admit it!) You will require your own legal counsel to evaluate the contract when you are serious about joining an office.

   I have personally seen the percentage of compensation paid to associates range from 15 to 42%!!! It is my PERSONAL OPINION that an equitable recompense in most offices is in the 30 to 32% range. (My associate is paid 30%.) The percent should always be based on collections. To pay for production creates a potential nightmare situation.

   Let's say a new associate has three hours open and an emergency patient who has never before been to the office is seen with a toothache. The young doctor may advise the patient that to keep the tooth will require a root canal, post and crown. The patient asks if they can do that today? The young dentist knows the schedule is open and says sure! Three hours later the young dentist has created $1,000 in production!

But the stuff hits the fan when the senior dentist, who pays for all the materials plus the associate's salary, learns nothing was ever collected and no financial arrangements were made with this patient. The associate has made a nice sum of money based on production, but when the patient doesn't pay, the money comes from the senior doctor's own wallet. Believe me, in the long run, everyone loses.

If the associates understand they receive nothing if the patient doesn't pay for their care, this type of problem should never happen . . . at least not more than once.

Also please bear in mind, selecting an office where you'll be busy is much more essential than the percentage of collection you receive; 42% of $1,000 a week is not as good a deal as 30% of $3,000 collected. It is the **documented growth of the practice** and the **new patient flow** that will tell if you will be busy in any given practice. Also, if the senior doctor wishes to add a dentist because of cutting back time in the office, much of the care this doctor previously performed will be shifted to you. If the owner is young and aggressive, you may have to fight for patients, and you won't win many of those battles.

8. *KEY POINT!!!* Ask to be given a copy of the most current three years' profit and loss statements, prepared by an accountant for the business. It may prove necessary to personally pay your own accountant to help you accurately digest these vital facts and figures. You are looking for trends, hopefully growth ones. Have both production and collection increased in the last three years, and if so by how much? If there hasn't been an increase, does the doctor have an explanation for this fact?

   For example, if the office went from two doctors to one, or if the senior doctor has significantly cut back on days in the office, you can't reasonably expect to see growth.

> You should also ask for an EXACT COUNT (do not accept an estimate) of new patients seen in each of the last three years. Entering a practice in decline is likely to prove hazardous to your financial health!

There is a lot of information you will absorb just by being in the office. How do you like the look of the office? Is it busy? Does the staff seem pleasant and efficient? Are they happy? (Because if they aren't, you won't be.) Do you feel comfortable with the doctor? Some folks we just seem to relate to, and others not. Does your spouse share your feeling?

What condition is the equipment in that you'll be using? You don't have to be an expert to tell how it looks. Did you meet the chairside you will be working with? Did you like each other?

As you travel home, discuss the community itself. Does it contain the essential requirements you demand to be happy? Would you be proud to show your friends and family around town? Is this a place you would choose to raise your family? Were the people you met friendly? Does the community show signs of growth? The basic question you're trying to answer: IS THIS A PLACE WHERE YOU **BOTH** CAN FIND JOY?

Next review your overall impressions of the office, doctor and staff. What are the concerns you have? What real positives can you see? As always, record your impressions.

And lastly we evaluate the critical numbers! If there is no patient load for you, nothing else matters, as you'll soon be leaving the office. If, in the last two years, collection has gone from $300,000 to $340,000, that is a 13% growth and very impressive! It is difficult for a doctor working alone to collect much in excess of $500,000 per year (although some definitely accomplish this task and a precious few greatly exceed it). It may not be fair to expect much growth from this elevated level, but new patient flow should continue to rise.

As a number to hang your hat on, the Iowa State Dental Association informs me the average dental office in our state sees approximately 120 new patients annually. Doctor Long and I combined see 300 to 400 new patients per year. This will give you an idea of how the office you are evaluating compares.

Let me leave you with this thought. If you start an office from nothing and grow at 120 patients a year, how long until you are busy? I would estimate about 1,000 patients to be the minimum needed for a one-doctor office to be working steadily. Our office has about 5,000 active patients and another 5,000 inactive (i.e.: They have been there and left. They may have moved, died or just got mad and took a hike).

Your circuits may well be suffering overload from too much sensory stimulation. Let's back away from this intense analysis for a moment and allow me to share my personal feelings and experience concerning solo versus group practice. You may still at this juncture be considering both, but the moment of definitive choice quickly approaches.

## Chapter Seven

# The Pros and Cons of a Small Group Practice

We examined the question of whether you as an individual are best suited by temperament and disposition for a solo or group practice arrangement in Chapter Three, just before we began our critical value clarification work.

Since that time we've dealt almost exclusively with the concerns that arise when we are selecting a community in which to practice and evaluating an existing practice as a possible business opportunity. (My redundant use of the word "business" is an attempt to create an awareness of the fact that when you leave school you indeed enter the world of BUSINESS—no more or no less.)

Our focus will soon switch to the considerations necessary to buy an existing office outright. This process involves many of the same basic premises as selecting a practice to join entails, with one very significant difference: To buy a practice you must determine its fair price.

We'll also soon be shifting our focus to what is required to start a practice from scratch . . . a daunting task in any times, but more so today with the higher level of debt most graduates have—yet still eminently possible.

Before we commence those dialogues, I'd like to share with you my most personal feelings concerning small group practices. Clearly understand that what follows are merely my thoughts based on my experiences, and not universal truths. But I believe, in combination with the information you've absorbed so far, augmented by your own value clarification process, that this information centered on my own 20-plus years of dental practice experience will prove valuable to you.

Please be aware that despite my greatest efforts at rigorous fairness, everything I write is from the prospective of one who has employed associates, but never been one. If you sense an unconscious bias, forgive me, but I believe that understanding the situation and the mind-set of the owner-dentist will be a tremendous asset to those of you seeking associate positions.

After 11 years of solo practice, I made a decision to select an associate to join our dental team. That decision was made in 1985. Now, two of us practice in what, for so many years, was just my office. The years which followed my decision to add other providers to our practice have contained many delights, but also not a few horrors. I am personally totally committed to a group concept and would never consider solo practice again. Yet daily, I'm aware of all the extra problems a group practice entails, and often reflect back with "my" staff on the good old days—when it was just us.

I'd like to share with you in as evenhanded a manner as possible the advantages and disadvantages of a small group practice. I think, next to marriage, the choice to enter group practice is the biggest decision most professionals make. Let's take a serious look on both sides of the group practice fence.

Forgive the necessary redundancy, but the critical, first step for any doctor is to *clarify why he/she would consider a group*. For me personally, the pressure of solo practice became just too great. In 1985, our office was collecting $40,000 per month, had 5000 active patients (by actual record count), and often saw 10 or more emergency patients a day. I felt I had maximized my own productive capabilities—with five fully equipped operatories and an excellent, experienced staff of seven—but I still couldn't keep abreast of the patient demand. The choices were:

a) Get some help or

b) Turn patients away.

I returned from a week of March skiing in Colorado to confront a document hanging on my office wall. The fateful list contained the names of 45 people who had emergency dental problems. We had a completely full schedule for the upcoming week. The emergency patients were in pain and already displeased at having been forced to wait a week for me to return.

In the course of the following five days we treated approximately twenty additional emergency patients who contacted us during the week itself. The skiing had been lovely, but the 18-hour nonstop drive to Colorado and back had been long and fatiguing. I returned to my office worn out before my marathon of dental care even began. Somewhere in the course of that week I experienced a moment of epiphany: I REALLY NEED SOME HELP!

From the perspective of a young professional, just starting in the business of dentistry, reasons we've discussed to consider joining a group practice may include:

1. A lack of funds, or an oversupply of debt, making it financially difficult to begin your own practice.
2. A desire to have an experienced dentist available to help in the development of clinical and business skills.
3. A personal lack of interest in the business aspects of dentistry.

An established doctor may investigate the possibilities of adding an associate because:

1. They desire help in treating an excessive patient load,
2. Would value the sharing of overhead expenses to reduce those unrelenting pressures, or

3. To build a relationship with someone who one day will wish to buy all or a part of their practice, and thus free some equity capital for the owner. These and many more excellent reasons exist to consider a group practice.

Since I have chosen to work in a group practice setting, I'll begin with the pros, but I want to caution you that the cons are also compelling. Each doctor considering a group must evaluate all the factors we'll discuss, plus many more individual concerns I've not included in our discussion. He or she must assign a level of personal importance or weight to each factor based on his/her experiences and clarified values in an effort to make the best decision for the unique situation.

Let's consider the advantages to group practice:

## 1. More New Patients

With multiple providers we were forced by limited space (five operatories and 2000 square feet) to stagger our hours of patient care and to offer evening and Saturday appointment times.

The positive side of this change in our working hours was the added patient convenience created. *This single change in our office hours led to a 50 percent increase in new patient flow almost immediately after a second doctor joined our practice.* In Keokuk, families with both spouses working and people reluctant to take kids out of school found this added availability of our care very attractive. The presence of another doctor and added staff in the community also led to an increased awareness of our practice which further enhanced new patient flow.

Over the years as our office size has varied from two to three doctors, by some alchemy I can't precisely describe, the flow of new patients has changed in relation to the number of dentists employed at any given moment in our office. While I am unable to explain it, all of us are grateful for this occurrence. Maybe it's similar to the movie, *Field of Dreams*—if you provide the capacity for care, they will come.

## 2. Lower Fixed Overhead

Dentists as a group seem loath to work with numbers. Yet, we are well above average in our training and ability to do so. Maybe our profession's long monopoly status has made us wasteful and lazy. **No business can function efficiently without understanding the facts of the enterprise.** To run a dental office as a profitable business the math must be done.

When I break my actual office figures down for you and analyze them, pay your most strict attention. You must develop this ability to understand the arithmetic of practice if you desire profitability. In today's market this ability is **ESSENTIAL.**

We needed to make almost no changes to our office physical plant when we added an associate. The cost of our heating, cooling, phones, business insurance (not malpractice, of course) and rent stayed pretty much the same. In 1986, our office overhead percentage dropped from 65 percent (as a solo practitioner with a staff of seven), to 58 percent with two doctors and nine staff working in our office. Our average office production went from $40,000 to $60,000 per month.

So many little changes occurred in the transition to a multi-doctor practice that it's difficult to establish a precise figure as our fixed overhead savings, but I think it's fair to say rent, utilities and some insurance are cut in half (or into thirds, during the years we had a three-doctor office) and many other expenses are reduced to a lesser extent.

For example, in 1986, as we discussed, we went from seven staff members to nine after the addition of our first associate, while our collected dollars went from $40,000 to $60,000 monthly. Working alone, we had produced $5,700 per staff member per month. With an associate's production added, we increased to $6,600 per staff member per month. The bottom line, and to me the biggest factor of the group concept, is *more net dollars are left to share among all the doctors involved in the practice.*

I can't overstress this vital point. The total dollars brought into the office increases, while the percentage of overhead drops. This gives a double accelerator effect to our net, as both increased production and collection, as well as reduced percentage of overhead, lead to an increase in my old friend NET PROFIT.

To use the figures quoted above from our first year with an associate as an example, we went from $40,000 collection per month average and 65% overhead—and thus a $14,000 per month net—to $60,000 per month collections at 58% overhead, or a $25,200 per month net.

Granted, this profit is now split between two doctors.

How an associate is compensated will depend on the geographic area in which you reside, your own philosophy and many other variables—but let's examine these numbers in two other ways. Say your associate produces $20,000 per month (as ours did) and you pay him 30% of the collected total (this was the original contract figure for our first associate). Thus his salary for that month is $6,000 (30% of $20,000). The practice net was $25,200 and less the $6,000 associate earnings, the senior doctor's net is $19,200. *The owner's net has increased $5,200 dollars per month, or $62,400 per year, and your production and time spent chairside have stayed the same.*

Have you "stolen" the money that your poor associate earned by the sweat of the—shall we say, brow? Let's examine the numbers again. You have reduced overhead (as good managers are wont to do) by seven percent. Seven percent of $60,000 is $4,300. So, all but $900 of your increased profits comes from your managerial expertise by reducing your costs of doing business and not from the production of the additional dentist.

I feel this $900 is well earned by the senior dentist. He/she has provided the patient load, the trained staff, as well as the philosophy and vision of success. It is he/she who has made the effort to search and hire the proper person for the office. All these accomplishments make the owner deserving of a reward. To employ a skilled and experienced office manager would be an expense at least double this $900 per month figure the office owner (I) received in our example.

One last point: This additional profit continues month after month, unless the associate improves in skills. Then it **increases.**

## 3. Added Cash Flow

Adding new equipment and services becomes much less a financial burden due to the accelerated production capabilities of a multi-provider office. Adding a Panorex, intraoral camera or computer system, as well as continuing education expenses, are more affordable due to the increased cash flow. As the new additions in equipment or services available are used for more hours and benefit more patients, they also increase profitability to a greater extent than possible in a solo office.

In a solo practice, some of these needed and welcomed additions are difficult to justify financially. It is virtually impossible for a single doctor's office to keep pace with a group when it comes to updated facilities or marketing efforts. The group is simply making a double or triple return over the solo practitioner on every practice-enhancing investment.

## 4. Mini-specialization

In our community of 13,000, the only specialty support is that of a full-time orthodontist and an oral surgeon who visits town every Tuesday. I used to do a lot of procedures of a specialty nature to accommodate people. (Most specialists in our area don't have expanded hours, so a trip to their office could mean a lost day of work as well as travel expenses for our patient.) Often, these procedures were stressful to me and I felt they would have been performed at a higher level of quality, with much less attendant effort, by a much more qualified specialist.

Whether by luck or design, in our current group, we each have unusual skills and/or interests in a different specialty area of dental practice. (Actually, Doctor Long has skills, I have interest.) This allows each of us to spend more time performing the sub-specialties of dentistry we most enjoy. We are allowed to concentrate our energies and talents in those areas we prefer, and thus are able to provide the patients with a better service based on our expanded experience and studies. Our increasing level of knowledge and skill in our particular areas of expertise allows us to work more quickly and efficiently. This increase in quality of care justifies an increase in our fee for that service. Of course, both increased efficiency and a higher fee add to our NET.

As an example, I no longer remove teeth—a job I did reluctantly for years but never enjoyed. This saves patients from my less than complete mastery of the art of exodontia. It keeps me from having to do procedures I dislike almost to the point of phobia. It also means another member of our group—who for reasons mysterious to me enjoys removing teeth—gets to provide more of this service to our patients. Of course, as his skills exceed mine in this area, the treatment is completed much more quickly. We make more money, and few patients complain they wish we had pulled their tooth more slowly.

Much of the treatment I had referred out in the past now stays in our office. Some of it, if the provider is skilled and efficient in that particular area, is very lucrative. The patients much prefer to be seen in our office rather than to be referred to an office they are unfamiliar with that is usually some distance away. (This is called the "better the devil you know" syndrome.)

### 5. Peer Review

We all are human and fail at times in our "practice" of dentistry. It is still uncomfortable when one of the caring, committed fellow doctors I've worked with points out a procedural shortcoming to me, or I to him. We do so because of our commitment to our patients and because we know this outside evaluation helps us to grow professionally. Perhaps it shouldn't matter, but knowing my friends and fellow dentists will see those crown margins or endo fills increases my effort to do my best.

As admittedly uncomfortable as it is to have an associate point out a less than perfect result to you, the prospect of a peer review committee or (God forbid) an attorney making the same point is much less appealing.

## 6. Mutual Support

"Nobody knows the troubles I've seen"—except another dentist. Staff, even your spouse or children may be concerned and sympathetic, but no one else **knows**. It can be a great help to have a friend right in the office who really does understand that at times, even your mightiest efforts aren't good enough.

Emotionally another doctor has complete empathy, as they have been precisely in your shoes in the past. Physically they may be able to step in and assist in a clinical situation that is progressing from bad to worse, despite all your efforts. What we do for a living is lonely work. It helps to have a friend close at hand. This friend is not only committed to you emotionally, but your futures are tied financially as well. I can't imagine a more dedicated advocate than your own associate.

All this discussion has been pitched to associates and not partners, for the simplest of reasons: I have never had a partner. I also never will. No amount of money would ever tempt me to give up control of a practice I have devoted over 20 years of my life to developing. I would certainly sell a part of my incorporated office, but never a controlling interest. If your interest lies in partnerships, you may need an additional book.

I don't mean to sound judgmental concerning partners. Partnership may work wonderfully well for some people and in certain situations. Great for them! But I'm a leader. I don't like decisions made in committee. For me collecting all possible staff input, and then deciding for myself what is best, is the only system I'll consider.

On the negative side of group practice, two things are of major concern to me. After years of effort, I fear that for me at least, these may be problems not to be solved, but to be endured.

## 1. Loss of Shared Vision

The larger the group, the harder it is to share a clear purpose or vision. As you know, our office spent a year writing our purpose. This was completed before we became a multiple-doctor practice. For years, our purpose was the epicenter of our practice. Personally, it still reflects what gives the practice of dentistry meaning to me. I'm not sure I can claim that all of our staff is committed to this vision today.

A plaque inscribed with our purpose still hangs on the wall of every room in our office. We still read this document before each staff meeting. I'd dearly love to tell you all of us are committed to it, but sadly, I can't. Of all the problems we'll discuss, this, to me, is by far the greatest and the one I seem least able to solve. The sense of teamwork gained from common values is no longer as strong.

As the number of people involved in our group grows, it seems inevitable that the strength of these values be diminished. We have had doctors in our office who were almost scornful of our creed. At first such an attitude was puzzling to me. Part of the reason they chose to join our office was our success. Our PURPOSE played a critical role in our accomplishments. Now, I believe I see that though they admired the success we have achieved, they were also threatened by it. They have a need to assert their independence. I'm afraid it is all too human to belittle or even attack that which you perceive to be stronger or greater than you.

Logically I feel they should study what we have done, and emulate the parts that are consistent with their own values. Realistically, I've never employed an associate doctor I felt attempted to do this. Of course, none of our beliefs or systems are forced on them. They are free to follow our ways or create their own. My personal philosophy and experience with life show me no other possible course of action to follow.

I'm sure there exist people clever enough to copy a winning concept. Unfortunately none of the five associates who have graced our office over the years has truly done so. I believe the need of ego to assert itself when it feels threatened is just too strong. If I were an associate in our practice, possibly I would do the same. (But I sure hope not.)

## 2. Loss of Control:

Maybe this is part of a loss of vision, but it was very hard for me (and I'm sure as hard for my associates) not to be *the* doctor; not to have all the staff and patients be *mine*. If the senior dentist wants an associate to stay, he must *give up some control of staff and patients*. He can be the team quarterback, but not the king of the office. I don't believe an outstanding doctor will choose to work in **your** office—it must become **his/hers**, too. This can't happen unless they are given the authority to make decisions on their own.

As I stated earlier, I want no partners. On the other hand, I allow my associates complete control over how they manage their part of our practice, as long as the quality of care we provide to our patients is not compromised. We use only the best dental materials, instruments and labs. All of the associate doctors have chosen to copy us in these matters. It is in the hours they work and the methods of interaction with patients and staff they adopt that their individualism is expressed.

All doctors and staff are required to attend and participate in our full office staff meetings. Most of the doctors have chosen not to participate in a morning clearing with their staff, or to review each patient's record before the day begins—as I do. I state these things only to give a full and honest report on the status of our office. I neither like nor agree with their choices, but in reality, they are just that . . . their choices.

I think they believe (or hope at least) that great success can be achieved without expending quite the effort we put in. How about you? Is there somewhere you go looking for a free lunch?

The minor frustrations, but ones I feel we can someday control or eliminate, include:

## 1. Staff Conflict

It's true, as staff increases in size, conflict increases geometrically. Also, cliques start to develop, and sadly, people become loyal to "their" doctor. (Loyalty should be to "our" patients, but it doesn't always work that way.) We labor consciously and consistently on communication skills—we always have—and continue to devote a section of each staff meeting to a communication exercise (which we'll discuss fully in Chapter Thirteen), but these conflicts continue to be an annoyance.

### 2. More Frequent Mistakes

Job descriptions are less clear due to more people being involved in our projects. Also, with expanded hours, a person who begins a job (like study models or post-operative calls) is not always the one who finishes it. This opens the door for more errors. Communication lines become more muddled, so lab cases may not be sent promptly or post-op calls aren't made at all.

A lot of little oversights and errors occur with our current, multiple front-office people compared to when just one or two staff members performed everything. It is also easier for duplication of efforts to occur, such as two people calling the same patient to confirm a next day appointment. Similar complications seem inevitable as more people are involved in the same tasks.

### 3. Equipment Breakdowns

Due to expanded use of our facilities, we need more equipment repairs. It's not only the added expense, but not having a piece of equipment available when you need it is frustrating. Also, I get a little annoyed every time "my" chair is repositioned. Instead of everything being set just as I prefer, now constant minute adjustments are needed by each doctor. Occasionally, some needed supplies aren't ordered when they should be, or not replaced in their correct spot when they are received.

I guess the answer to these "little" things is a 4000-square-foot office with nine ops, but that eliminates the reduced overhead that, to me, is the biggest advantage of a group.

Each of you can add other concerns, I'm sure, but for me, these have been the major considerations involved in a group practice setting. However, the biggest variable will be your own personality. Recall the questions I encouraged you to ask yourself in Chapter Three: Do you enjoy working with others? Can you submerge your ego (it won't disappear, but for most of us it can be controlled) for the good of a team? Do you have an awareness of your own dominant personality type and is it compatible with group practice? With proper leadership, the financial advantages are great, as I think each year's *Dental Economics* survey comparing solo and group practice finances illustrates.

The pressures of dentistry can be decreased in a group environment for all the reasons we've discussed. But you'll have to look deep inside yourself to see if these benefits make tolerating the disadvantages worthwhile. I urge you to look **carefully** before you leap. A group practice started without careful planning can closely resemble a hasty marriage. Remember the old saw—"marry in haste, repent at leisure."

The economies of scale we discussed also come to play in a satellite office situation, with one small twist—they are reversed. That's right, now fixed overhead increases, and net is diminished. I haven't purchased a satellite office, so these comments are philosophical only, and not supported by personal experience. If you are tempted to pursue a second practice location, be certain you understand the overhead concerns we discussed here, as those same principles apply to a satellite. Be very sure of your decision before you act; as the "repent at leisure" part applies also. I believe you'll discover it's a whole lot easier to buy a dental practice than it is to sell it.

## Chapter Eight

# Purchasing a Practice

I've done all within my poor powers to assist you in reaching a decision whether to pursue group or solo practice opportunities. I've guided your search within for self-discovered answers. I've shared my own dental journey of over 20 years, and my resultant feelings on the subject with you. I suspect that, over the course of your long careers, a good many of you will find yourself in both a solo and group practice situation for some period of time.

Group practices have steadily grown in popularity since I first darkened my own office door. The most current ADA statistics I've seen reveal that 35% of current graduates begin their professional lives as participants in some form of multi-doctor situation.

One of the great powers—even if they be dark forces by our lights—that has fueled this trend is a steady 1% increase in annual overhead (or decrease in net!) that our profession has averaged in each year of the last decade. One percent may not seem significant, but a 10% reduction in profit for the same effort demanded has even our profession—so slow to react—looking for answers.

There seemingly is no end to this insidious downward pressure on our profession's profit margin. Apparently each doctor and each office must try to discover their own remedies to this malady as best they can. In the preceding chapter I did my best to demonstrate how a well-run group reduces overhead pressures, thus increasing net profit. While there are many strategies that can be employed to increase profits in any practice, the great overhead reduction available from a group setting is the most efficacious method to significantly increase overall practice net of which I am aware.

In the next chapters we will discuss:

1. How to purchase an existing practice—dealt with immediately.
2. What steps you must take to open an office on your own—covered in following chapters.

Much of the information we have already shared will prove useful no matter what practice venue you choose to pursue. Our beginning values clarification work is essential for all who seek success and joy, but will be most imperative for those hardy souls who choose to practice alone, as more frequent and critical decisions will be required of them, demanding a clearer understanding of themselves.

Likewise, the method whereby you identify an area, and then narrow this broad choice to a community you would choose to grow old in remains unchanged, whatever practice mode you select.

Also, a great deal of the practice evaluation for purchase process is identical to that done when considering an associate position. You still want to know the office reputation within the community. You must know if the staff are well trained, enjoy their jobs and wish to stay. Even a plan to transfer patients remains critical, but in a practice sale situation would involve a letter to each patient from the departing dentist, or perhaps her staying for a period of time to introduce the purchaser to the practice's patients.

The one quintessential difference that exists between the evaluation of a potential associateship and an office purchase is the hub upon which all business rotates: How to arrive at a fair price for the office you wish to purchase, and how to finance the acquisition.

Let's get one vital point crystal clear. When you buy an office the key asset you are purchasing is **INCOME FLOW.** Every practice's lifeblood comes from patients who seek your care. Anyone can buy dental equipment, but when you purchase an existing office, a flow of patients comes with the chairs, x-rays, and assorted dental hardware. If this is not so, you may as well build your own office exactly as you choose, rather than accepting an office built by another dentist based on his or her personal dreams.

The basic places we look to identify a practice for sale remain the same as during our search for an associateship—ADA, state and other dental journal ads, dental schools, dental sales representatives, state and local dental societies—with one big difference. Now PRACTICE BROKERS play a much more central role. The reason for that is simple: MONEY. As is the case with most real estate, a dental office is sold for a fee, and sales commissions are how practice brokers make their living.

Brokers are **hired by the practice owners or sellers.** That is who pays them and that is whom they work for, despite how they present themselves or how it may appear to the buyer. Never lose track of this basic fact. There is nothing venial about their relationship—this is simply the reality of the situation. The deception comes into play if the broker leads you—the buyer—to believe that they are on your side. You must flip them over (figuratively only, please!) to see which side has all the butter. (It's the practice seller's side!)

IF YOU CAN'T CALCULATE THE APPROXIMATE VALUE OF A PRACTICE ON YOUR OWN IT WILL COST YOU DEARLY! Several practices in our area have been sold to "bigger fools than first bought them." One local office now boasts the fourth dentist-owner since I've moved to Keokuk. The other three all gave up and sold out. At least the price keeps dropping. I evaluated the office for one of the dentists that left (number three, I believe) and felt I could use it as a satellite and be busy, at best, two days a week. The price asked was roughly double my estimate of the office's value, and the exact amount remaining on the failing practice's bank note. (Life is indeed replete with coincidences.) I declined the invitation to be the next holder of this struggling practice's bank note.

I don't think it is happenstance that all four of the doctors who have purchased this practice have been new dental school graduates. Welcome to our world—the business jungle of buyer beware!

Let's begin this portion of our journey with the assumptions that we've located a community we wish to call home. We can hardly wait to show our parents around! We have visited a practice for sale and are positively impressed. The staff seem very efficient and pleasant. They like their jobs and very much wish to stay within the office. The practice is busy and productive. The owner is retiring, and you like her. She seems to truly enjoy the office, patients and staff.

The practice owner has never bought or sold an office during the course of her career, so we seem poised to begin the dance of the blind, with perhaps the "altruistic" broker as dance master.

In small communities at least, even attorneys and accountants may have no experience with the sale of a professional business. AND SIMPLE RULES OF THUMB TO VALUE PRACTICES DON'T WORK. You must educate yourself concerning this process or suffer the consequences of your ignorance!

Permit me to walk you through the best source of information on valuing a practice I've found—and I've read more than I wish to on the subject. But first, allow me to clearly state that I have never bought or sold a practice. I have painstakingly calculated the value of my own office at the request of one of my previous associates who was considering buying a share of the professional corporation that is my practice. I have also "worked the numbers" on three area offices that were for sale when I was approached to see if I had any interest in purchasing them. I gave each practice the serious consideration I would give any business venture (and that's damn serious for me). I also worked very diligently when estimating a value for my office, as we were dealing with my business, my life and MY MONEY!

So I have some "book learning" about the topic, but have never been bloodied in actual battle. There is a big difference between reading about something and doing it, and I want all of you to be aware of that. I am always on the lookout to purchase a small office at the right price—I think a wise practice acquisition can be a great investment for a sharp businessman-dentist, and often envy urban practices for the relatively wide variety of practice purchase opportunities available to them—but I've never bought another office.

Each of you who is serious about buying an office—in addition to the information you are about to digest—should read the reference I will cite in a moment to feel at least minimally prepared before undertaking such a critical task.

Good news! The book is easy to read and a concise 50 pages! It uses the "how to eat an elephant" school of practice valuation—one bite at a time. There are many examples and workbook pages to be sure even the math-adverse (me foremost among you) can understand their points.

The book is published by the ADA and can be yours for a few dollars. It is entitled *Successful Valuation of a Dental Practice, Volume Two.* It can be purchased by writing to the main ADA headquarters at:

American Dental Association
211 East Chicago Ave.
Chicago, Illinois 60611
or by phoning the ADA main office at 1-800-621-8099.

Let me point out one last critical premise before we begin our study of this worthy resource. Both the buyer and the seller want and need to establish a fair price for the practice, but neither may know how. They both wish an equitable price, not because all dentists are noble—that's just a coincidence—but because they understand that if both parties don't win, everyone loses.

If the buyer pays too much, she may go broke and dump the practice back on the seller, who is just really beginning to love the new life in Arizona. Suddenly, the previous owner discovers the office payments have stopped and starts considering moving back to Iowa for the winter to reopen the practice until the office can be sold again. What a fine kettle of fish that is! (Note: Only the broker, who received the full commission, is happy. They get their money first and keep it no matter what the eventual outcome of the sale, and they are usually paid an even larger commission if the practice sells for more.)

Allow me to mention one last essential advantage of the aforementioned ADA booklet from which much of the following material is drawn. This ADA source comes to you without bias. It is written from the perspective of neither buyer nor seller, unlike much of the other available information on practice purchases. You will find, as you journey through your careers, that unbiased information is a precious and rare commodity.

Let's jump bravely into the dead middle of the fray and deal with the issue of how to establish A FAIR PRICE FOR AN OFFICE.

Price is determined by what someone is willing to pay for the commodity. I have a No. 2 lead pencil worth $1,000, or at least I do if you'll pay me $1,000 for such a fine writing instrument. Of course, the buyer and seller must agree that the final price is fair to both or there will be no sale. (This may explain why my pencil sales have been off lately, despite their darling canary yellow color.)

I believe, for a dental practice to be sold and have both parties feel they have been treated equitably, the final price must allow the purchaser (you!) to:

1. Meet all office expenses,

2. Draw a realistic, livable salary and
3. Eliminate the purchase debt in a reasonable period of time (from 4 to 6 years, as we'll see). The above description must be true if we are to maintain that a fair practice value has been established. Now that we have a general target firmly in our sights, we can get to work determining how a specific dollar office value can be derived.

Let's discuss the most common reasons a practice may need to be valued. There are many more such occasions than one might assume on the basis of cursory thought. Seeing the importance and required frequency of such a valuation may make this exercise a bit more meaningful to every reader.

## A practice must be valued:

1. When the practice is to be sold—the focus of our current discussion.
2. When a *portion* of the practice is to be sold. All of you who may one day buy or sell a partnership share or stock in a professional corporation need to gather around and listen up too.
3. When considering a future buy-in for an associate. **THIS IS A CRITICAL POINT FOR MY READERS TO CONSIDER NOW.** Many associate candidates plan to "someday" buy into the office they select in which to begin their careers. Often the owners employ the associate with this same long-term understanding on their part. Unfortunately, just when both doctors agree that things are going very well and sit down to discuss a permanent relationship and establish a purchase price, they may find they are far apart on their individual estimates of the practice's value. Often this leaves each party feeling poorly used by the other and bitter. A pleasant association that could have proven beneficial and profitable to both parties is destroyed.

   **For those of you joining a practice as an associate with plans of possibly purchasing all or a part of that practice at some**

**future point, it is IMPERATIVE that you and the owner have a mutually agreed-upon FORMULA in place, before your associateship begins, from which you may easily determine the value of the office at a later date.**

Certainly, it is impossible to attempt to set a precise value on an office at some unspecified future date. But an agreement can be reached—using the information available in this chapter—that will define the method by which the final price will be determined, leaving you to merely plug the agreed-upon current numbers into your mutually accepted formula when both parties concur it is time to do so.

4. The practice must be valued if you seek a loan, for any reason—office expansion, adding new equipment, remodeling. This information is required by banks in their efforts to judge the sagacity of loaning money to any business. Dental offices seldom go bankrupt and make excellent loan prospects, but the failure to achieve bank financing by dentists is often caused by the bank's indelible perception that they are *not dealing with a businessman!* Requesting a loan be made without having established a clear value of the asset that will be the loan's collateral is an example of extremely unbusinesslike behavior.

5. In case of divorce. This is a far too common cause of asset valuation in our society generally and our profession specifically. Divorce court does not lie on the road to joy. How often do busy doctors sacrifice for "success," ignoring or abandoning those they care about in their great effort to achieve, only to finally live in misery as a result? (The correct answer is way too often!) **Such an outcome is the result of unclear values and a failure to understand the relationship between wisdom and joy. The readers of this book have no such excuses!**

So the need for valuation of a practice is a more common and important part of our BUSINESS than one might have assumed at first blush.

Let's next briefly consider the TERMS OF A SALE. Here we deal with the most basic of investment truths—the relationship of risk and reward and the concept of the time-use cost of money. For any investment, the greater its risk, the higher the reward that must be offered to the investor to convince him or her to buy the asset.

For example, if an ultra-safe U.S. Government bond pays a 7% yield, a bond of low quality (say a B-rated corporate bond for those of you who possess some familiarity with investing) may have to pay a 10% yield to induce investors to take the EXTRA RISK THIS INVESTMENT REPRESENTS.

In the same fashion, a government bond (considered the world's safest investment) that matures in one year may pay a 5% yield, while a 3-year government bond returns a 7% yield. The longer the time frame, the greater the inherent uncertainty, thus the more risk and the higher the yield offered in response. Investment risk must be compensated for by increased rewards or the investors won't make the deal. Get the picture?

But, how does this affect the sale of a dental office? The universal principles of risk-reward remain identical in any business venture.

If you pay for an office with 100% cash, the price of the practice should be reduced to its lowest possible level, as all risk to the seller (once the check clears the bank at least) is gone. If you finance your office purchase over a short term (thus reducing investment risk) with a large down payment, the total price you pay should be significantly less than if you wish the seller to personally hold a 15-year note with little or none of the buyer's money paid up front. Can you comprehend how risk, and its cousin time, will raise or lower the price of the same office by variations in their themes?

Also imperative in any office sale is that WHAT YOU ARE PURCHASING MUST BE PRECISELY DEFINED. Does the price include accounts receivable? (Money owed the selling doctor by patients already treated.) What about dental and office supplies, cabinets, furniture? Every item to be sold must be clearly identified so a fair price can be established and misunderstandings avoided.

I'm familiar with a situation where an office was sold and the proud new owner came in Monday morning, only to find all of the cabinets had been torn out of the walls and removed. The cabinets had been specially built for the seller and he felt they remained his, just as the removable equipment was. The buyer assumed, since the cabinets were attached to the walls, they would stay as a permanent part of the office. Cabinets are expensive and these were both unhappy dentists, each feeling badly mistreated by the other. Such essential details must be clarified.

A specific date on which the value of the office will be determined (Valuation Date) must also be set. "The office was found to have a value of $240,000 as of 1 January, 1995," is the way any office valuation must read.

## Valuation Assumptions

Listed here are the basic conditions that are assumed as standard when an office is sold. If any of these facts isn't so, that information must be clearly stated and the price adjusted to reflect this altered situation.

1. All liabilities of the practice are paid in full by the seller. This would include debt on the office, back taxes due, or any other future liability coming due against the business. If any such debts do continue to exist, they must be reflected in a reduction of the office sale price.
2. All information provided by the seller must be complete and honest. Failure of full and open disclosure could lead to the issue being settled in court.

   Let me buttress this point with a personal example. On one of the offices I have considered purchasing, the seller and I had reached a tentative agreement on price. All that remained was the clarifying of a few minor details, and the office was mine. My staff and I personally visited this office to inventory the patient records and determine that the number given us as active patients was accurate. (We'll describe this process carefully in a few pages.) Our own count showed the number of current patients represented to us by this dentist and his broker to be DOUBLE the actual number of active charts.

I had accepted this number on faith alone up to this point, and had, on the basis of this fact, spent a lot of time and energy evaluating the practice. When the discovery of the accurate number of active patients was made, I broke off the sale, and the doctor and I did not part as friends. Had I not discovered this deception until after the sale, we would have undoubtedly ended up in court.

. A COVENANT NOT TO COMPETE IS INCLUDED IN THE SALES AGREEMENT. This is an essential, yet complex part of any office sale. In a noncompetitive agreement, the seller agrees not to open a dental office within an agreed-upon distance (which may be miles in the country or blocks in the city) for an agreed-upon length of time (measured in years).

These covenants have been overturned in court as representing restraint of trade. If the terms and penalties attached to them are perceived by the court as too strict, the non-competition clause may be thrown out completely. Yet, without such an agreement, or with one too lenient in terms, the selling dentist could open a new office a block away from the one just sold and the buyer would lose most or all of the patients purchased.

Recently in our little town, a small used car lot was sold. The seller immediately opened a new lot directly across the street! (Obviously no non-competition clause was in the sales contract.) It was a much bigger and more impressive business than the one just sold—undoubtedly financed by cash from the sale of the old lot. In a matter of months the seller had taken back the old lot too, as the new buyer went broke.

I personally know of three dental offices that have gone to court over non-competition agreements. Getting this done correctly requires expert legal assistance, and is critical!

4. No peer review or legal action is pending against the office, or if any is in process, that fact must be clearly disclosed.
5. The seller will assist the buyer in the transition to new office ownership by remaining and introducing the new owner to the office's existing patient population. If this isn't the case, the practice's price should be reduced to reflect it. A general dentist will usually agree to stay for two to six months. For a specialty practice the normal transition time is one to two years, due to their reliance on general dentists' referrals.
6. The extent of any office contract with capitation plans should be revealed. As we've discussed, these can conceivably have a significant negative impact on profit margin.

Let's now take a look at what data you, your accountant, attorney and/or practice appraiser must obtain in order to establish the value of a practice. Hang with me on the information that follows. Much of it probably won't be completely clear if you have had no practice experience. I'll do my best to briefly describe each term, but you'll need the help of some or all of the professionals listed above (accountants, attorneys, dental company representatives) to complete a practice valuation. They will be totally familiar with each of the following items and be able to fill in any gaps in your own knowledge base.

## Financial Information

1. A balance sheet showing assets and liabilities of the office.
2. Copies of the practice's last three years' income tax returns.
3. Year-to-date income figures (unless you are fortunate enough to be considering a practice precisely at year's end) to assure you the practice's level of income hasn't altered since the year-end data was reported.

4. Estimates from TWO dental supply companies as to the value of existing equipment. (Two independent estimates should be more accurate than one.) These should be itemized for each piece of equipment and include the date each was purchased and the original price.
5. Cost of all leasehold improvements and the date they were performed. (Leasehold improvements are actions taken to enhance the office space itself, such as new carpet, wallpaper, plumbing, wiring, etc.)
6. Estimate of the value of all dental supplies on hand.
7. Total office production for the last three years broken down by provider (i.e., what income came from hygiene, and the total production from each doctor in the office) as well as broken down by months.
8. Total collections for the last three years reported by months also.
9. Total of accounts receivable and their aging. (Recall, accounts receivable are money owed the office by patients. Aging tells how much money has been owed for how long. Let's say an office has $30,000 in total accounts receivable; $10,000 of this debt is from the most current month, another $10,000 occurred over the last 60 days and the remaining $10,000 is owed for 90 days or more. THE LONGER MONEY IS DUE YOU THE LESS LIKELY YOU ARE TO COLLECT IT, SO THE VALUE OF THE DEBT DECREASES. (Yes, Virginia, some folks won't pay you!)
10. The amount of accounts written off in the last three years. (This is money patients owe you that you realize will never be paid and just dropped from the books in resignation.)
11. A monthly itemized breakdown of all office expenses over the last three years.

## Patient and Service Information

1. Total number of ACTIVE PATIENTS—usually defined as patients seen in the last 12 to 24 months. The way I establish this figure is to go into the office and with the help of a ruler, measure two feet of files. Then I go through each record of this random two feet and determine if the patients have been in the office over the last 24 months. Let's assume I find a total of 100 records in this two-foot section and 60 of these records meet our definition of active patients. I then measure the total feet of records to find the number of active patients in the practice.

   This is critical, as an older office could have records on file of patients that have been deceased for five years! (Recall my story about the office I ALMOST BOUGHT.) You must perform this record inventory yourself. NEVER ENTRUST THIS JOB TO THE BROKER OR SELLER, AS IT IS PRECISELY THESE ACTIVE PATIENTS YOU ARE PURCHASING THE PRACTICE TO OBTAIN.

   In our example, assume we measured a total of 60 feet of files filled with records belonging to the office. In our survey of 2 feet, we found 100 files, of which 60 were deemed active. Sixty total feet divided by our 2-foot sample = 30; 30 times 60 active patients per 2 feet gives us a total of 1,800 active patients.

2. Number of new patients seen each month for the last three years. I consider a new patient anyone who had a complete dental examination, but not just an emergency visit. You'll also need to break them down by adult and child new patient exams. Adult patients need greater amounts of care, so while you welcome the children into your office, mature new patients are more valuable.

3. Description of any contractual obligations of the office, such as the infamous IPOs, PPO or capitation plans.

4. The length of time each provider is scheduled or booked ahead with patient appointments. (PROVIDERS are all who care for

patients directly—basically each doctor and hygienist.) This information indicates how busy the office currently is.

5. Effectiveness of recall system. If there are 1800 patients active (to use our previous example) and your survey determines the hygienist saw 900 patients last year, only 50% of the patients were seen on recare. A higher percentage of patients actively involved in the recare system increases the office's value.

## Practice Facilities

1. Total square footage of office.
2. Number of current staff, job description, date of first employment, beginning and current salary and hours worked per year.
3. Copy of office lease.
4. Number of years the dentist has practiced in the community.
5. Number of days and hours each provider sees patients.
6. Future intent of the owner. Will they stay in the office to introduce the buyer, and if so for how long?

I hope most of these terms are clear to you. As I said, you must have skilled help to analyze this data, and these advisors can help you understand these vital facts.

Now that we comprehend what information we must acquire to accurately value an office, let's examine how the actual valuation process takes place.

## Chapter Nine

# Practice Valuation

We've set the table and the meal has been prepared. Every piece of information we will require to attach a dollar price to the practice we've set our heart on has been described and defined. Now it's time to sit down, tuck in our napkin and dig in. Let's see precisely how we go about valuing a dental practice.

In the preceding chapter we mentioned that "rule of thumb" office valuations aren't accurate enough to be of any value in the complex task before us. I neglected to state exactly what these digited devices were! Rude of me, but it's a part of the problem every writer has to face: You just can't explain everything at once. At least here we have a wrong that can be easily righted.

By rule of thumb I mean quick, easy ways to assign an office a price. If you read even a little of the literature on office valuation, there are several prominent shortcut practice valuation methods mentioned. Among them:

1. A practice is worth 100% of the last full year's gross collected dollars.

   If a practice gross is $400,000 with an 80% overhead, is it worth as much to you as an office grossing $400,000 with a 50% overhead? Didn't think so. The $120,000 difference in profit should have some impact on an office's value.

2. An office is worth the price of a similar office recently sold in the same geographic area.

   In Keokuk there have been two offices sold in the last twenty years. Not much help to me. But even if fifty were sold last year, why would their price have a bearing on the value of my **unique** office?

3. The intangibles are worth 100% of last year's NET INCOME.

   Let's delay our discussion of this subject until we deal with asset summary valuations later in this chapter and we more fully develop our understanding of office "intangibles."

While every practice valuation technique shares the same tragic flaw—there are a large number of subjectives involved—our three "thumb jobs" simply ignore too many variables. Why isn't quick and easy ever best?

Buying a practice may be the SINGLE BIGGEST EXPENSE OF YOUR LIFETIME. Usually you must go deeply into debt to accomplish this purchase. We don't want to overpay! If the shortcuts aren't accurate enough—and may be even grossly misleading—where does that leave us? In MY OPINION with two viable long cuts, both of which enable us to fairly value a practice.

## Capitalized Earnings

Remember in the previous chapter we defined a fair market price generically as one that allowed the buyer to meet office expenses, draw a reasonable salary and pay off debt within four to six years? Our capitalized earnings valuation method assures us all three of these essential criteria will be met.

Under this plan, the value of a practice is based on the EARNINGS POTENTIAL of the buyer. Three essential steps are involved:

1. Projecting the pre-tax earnings of the buyer. (This is money remaining after all practice expenses have been paid, but before the effects of taxes are considered.) The expenses will include such non-cash items as depreciation of equipment as well as the "reasonable salary" we will soon be describing.

2. Determining a capitalization (cap) rate. This is similar to the rate of return a buyer should expect on an investment, and as we've stressed, is very much affected by investment risk. A simple illustration of this concept may improve our comprehension. If investors can receive a safe and certain 7% return on a U.S. Government bond, they may not be tempted to try the more risky stock market arena unless they felt fairly certain they could receive a 12% return. In the investor's mind these two returns are EQUIVALENT, when adjusted for risk.

   For a dental practice a cap rate within the 18 to 25% range is considered normal. This means an investment can be paid off over a time period of four (at 25%) to six (at 18%) years.

3. So our formula for practice valuation is:

$$\text{PRACTICE VALUATION} = \frac{\text{WEIGHTED ANNUAL EARNINGS}}{\text{CAP RATE}}$$

   For example, if our office's projected earnings, after all expenses and a reasonable doctor's salary are removed, is $30,000 and we have determined a 25% cap rate to be equitable for the investment risk in this particular venture, the practice value would be:

$30,000/ 25% = $120,000.

I know . . . clear as mud! Don't panic, work with me here as we go back and clarify each term and figure individually.

First, it would seem easy enough to come up with average earnings figures. The annual profit and loss statement from our accountant has that total on the very bottom line for us! No sweat!

Not so fast. (I bet you were afraid of that.) We must go over each year's expenses and remove from the totals deductible items that are more personal than essential business expenses in nature. Only when these somewhat discretionary expenses are removed can a true earning figure be derived.

What type of expenses are we talking about? Did the owner spend excessively or foolishly? Not at all, but he or she was able—within the unyielding confines of the tax code—to use some business money to pay for personal preference items. These must be removed from the expense total and the office profit raised by this amount.

Examples of these personal items that business owners can choose to have paid with pre-tax business dollars but which are not essential office expenses include:

1. Office car
2. Charitable contributions
3. Continuing education costs
4. Personal insurance
5. Medical reimbursement
6. Pension plan
7. SALARY

What remains after removing items of this nature are the total dollars left in the practice when all of the required bills are paid, but no expenses of a personal nature are deducted.

Next, we must calculate our AVERAGE projected earnings by taking the last three years' incomes and assigning them a weight of 1, 2, 3. Assume the last three complete years' earnings records for the office we admire look like this:

1994......... $42,400
1993......... $40,600
1992......... $44,800

We triple the most recent year—1994—to give us a total of $127,200. We double 1993 for a $81,200 figure and weight 1992 at 1 for a $44,800 total. Add these figures and divide by six

($253,200/6), and you have the AVERAGE WEIGHTED EARNINGS of the last three years of $42,200.

Why a **weighted** average? To give the more recent years a larger impact. If we had used a simple average, 1992 has the same effect on earnings as 1994, yet clearly the more recent period is more germane to our interests.

We have referred to a "reasonable salary." The quotes are mine as I have no idea if there exists enough money to pay me "reasonably" to perform as I do in my office on my days there. But the ADA booklet unblinkingly states a reasonable salary to be 22 to 30% of gross revenue (collected dollars before ANY expenses are removed). If the office you're considering COLLECTED $500,000 last year, the salary range would be from $110,000 at 22% to $150,000 at 30%. I don't know who came up with these percentages, but they're as good a place to hang our hat as any. This somewhat arbitrary figure, and its wide range, is but one example of the subjective nature of these calculations.

To review, the top figure on our Step 3 practice value formula is weighted annual earnings. This is our income figure, minus all expenses to run the practice including reasonable salary, and placed in our three-year weighted average formula. Finance charges, or debt service aren't taken out of this total. Debt is not considered a cost of doing business, but rather a cost of getting into business. (The short version of this philosophical treatise is that you pay debt out of the stuff called profit after salary.)

The last figure we must create is our **cap rate**. This varies by our perception of risk involved in the purchase of the office we are considering. Another way to state this is that the stronger the practice, the more it is worth, so the LOWER OUR CAP RATE. Things that reduce the cap (and thus raise the practice value) include:

1. Staff that are skilled, pleasant and wish to stay. A history of low staff turnover during the life of the practice also enhances the office's value for reasons we've previously discussed.

2. A history of fast growth in collected dollars for the practice. If the practice has been declining in produced revenue—a not unusual scenario if the owner is nearing retirement—its value is decreased. An office that has been closed completely, possibly due to the death or disability of the owner-dentist, quickly loses value.
3. Large number of active patients, by your actual count.
4. High rate of new patients seen per month.
5. Stability of the practice in the community. Past multiple owners of an office is a cause for concern. (Why did they leave?) Such a history should reduce the office value.
6. Good office location, such as on a busy street, with lots of free parking. Is the practice located in a part of the community that is currently growing?
7. High percentage of recare effectiveness.
8. Excellent community reputation of the office.
9. Good (read high) fee structure. A low fee structure really hurts value, as retaining these below-average fees significantly reduces profit, yet raising the office's existing fees may mean losing some of the patients we have counted on for cash flow.
10. High percentage of patients with insurance.

There are many more such items that could be factored in, depending on the practice's unique situation. Use your judgment. But again, note the dilemma of how to precisely value each one. No matter what technique of valuation you choose, a great deal of judgment (guessing?) goes into the process.

Let's quickly review the capitalized earnings method of office valuation. We have calculated a weighted annual earnings for the last three years. This total is divided by the cap rate—your assessment of the quality of the office—to give us a final office value figure.

Let's use our arbitrary figure (made up) of $42,200 for our weighted average annual earnings. If we deem the subjective factors of the office to be very strong, we would assign a cap rate of 18%. This would indicate a growing, profitable office with an excellent physical plant and staff who wanted to remain in the practice. The price we would then pay to purchase the practice would be $42,200/18% = $234,000.

If, in our estimation, the intangibles are weak—the reverse of the strengths listed above—we would increase the cap rate to 25% and our practice value would drop to $42,200/25% = $168,800.

The great difficulty lies with the subjective determination of an adequate salary to some extent, but most essentially with arriving at an equitable cap figure. Despite these drawbacks, capitalized earnings is still the best office valuation system I have discovered, as it is based on the buyer's ability to pay for the office purchased.

I know this is confusing, even to experienced dentists. The 50-page ADA booklet I've mentioned makes it a lot more understandable. If this isn't clear now, turn back and review the material we've just covered before becoming even further bewildered.

## Asset Summary Method

Using this method of practice valuation we divide the office assets into two major categories, tangible and non-tangible. These main portions are then further sectioned into even smaller pieces, and each segment assigned a value. The office price is merely the total value of all the pieces. Simple, huh?

Tangible means objects you can touch. Valuing them is the easy part. The list includes such things as:

1. Dental equipment.
2. Leasehold improvements—like plumbing, carpeting, wall covering, electrical wiring.
3. Accounts receivable.
4. Office supplies.

And many more. These are commodities about which two reasonable people should be able to reach agreement concerning their value. Often, outside professional assistance will be required, such as using an accountant to figure the depreciation of items in the office and the help of supply company representatives to estimate the value of existing equipment and supplies.

Non-tangibles are things you can't touch (did I hear someone say . . . look out!?). They would include such valuable assets as:

1. Office goodwill.
2. Value of patient records.
3. Covenant not to compete.
4. Office telephone number.
5. Practice name.

These are much more **subjective** (that horrid word again!) by nature and thus harder to value. But never fear, the ADA booklet says their range should be between 1 to 1.5 of the last year's practice net. Great. In my office this would be a RANGE of $125,000!!! Something less than a surgical strike precision-wise.

They say that figures lie and liars figure. And adding up the estimated value of every paper clip is fine, but—if as is so often the case, the owner has to finance the sale—and if the buyer goes broke and the seller gets the office back—what difference does the accuracy of the value estimate make? In that scenario, "fair" doesn't make much sense as both parties suffer.

The ADA book covers Asset Summation in much greater detail. If that seems the path best suited for you to take, follow it. It is my PERSONAL OPINION ONLY that a value based on earning power, which is what the cap rate gives us, is fairer to both parties. It considers such essentials as, "If I can buy two offices for the same price, one collecting $1,000,000 last year with 80% overhead, the other collecting $400,000 with 50% overhead, which would I choose?" in a much more realistic manner.

I know this remains unclear. If you read the several books available in the ADA library on the subject, it will still be confusing. What can't be avoided is the subjective nature of so many of the essential ingredients of an office's value. You must perform many careful evaluations of offices you are considering on your own to begin to get a sense—through the process of comparison and your own growing experience—of relative value. Only personal experience can fill this void, and for someone with no practice experience, this is very challenging.

That's enough on practice valuation, but there remains some important information relating to practice sales in general I wish to discuss with you. First, two random bits of data:

Do you know why practices are placed on the market for sale in the first place? Only 30% are due to the death or retirement of the owner. The rest are caused by a doctor's decision to return to school or relocate.

It is usually easier to finance an existing practice purchase from the bank, as a stable stream of income can be fairly accurately projected. This is impossible to do when starting an office from scratch. But remember, you'll be living with an office design and equipment not of your choosing when you buy an existing office.

Let's finally look at the cast of supporting characters that play an ESSENTIAL ROLE in any office purchase.

## Practice Appraisers

These are individuals in the business of assigning an exact dollar value to a practice. They should be paid a **flat fee** for their services, not a percentage of the price of the office, to assure they have no vested interest in the final office value. The ADA suggests a fair fee for their service to be in the $1,200 to $4,000 range. They will review all the numbers we have been discussing, as well as visit the office personally to allow a more complete evaluation of the intangible items such as staff suitability, office location and decor.

**If you claim to be an office appraiser, you are one.** No specific license is required. That should serve as an adequate warning for all of us. How are we to protect ourselves? The main weapon at our command is to ask for a lengthy list of the appraiser's previous satisfied customers, including their home and office phone numbers. (If you're told releasing this list would violate the clients' confidentiality, and this just can't be done, I'd personally tell the appraiser to take a hike.) Then CALL THE PEOPLE ON THIS LIST! Find out if they were pleased with the appraiser. Were they pleasant, prompt and ACCURATE? Did they feel these people were trustworthy?

You may also ask appraisers if they have a history of defending their findings in court. Such experience could be a valuable asset in a worst case scenario of a business deal gone very wrong. Again, request references for this unfortunate situation. (Call and ask the appraiser's clients if they won, at least.)

Both the buyer and seller can have independent appraisals done. Certainly this is expensive, but gives you some protection not available if only the seller has the appraisal performed. This also looks more thorough and professional if you need bank financing.

## Attorney

They will be required in most practice transitions to draw up the actual contract of sale. Lawyers tend to prefer certain areas of the law, just as most dentists choose some specific area of dental practice they most enjoy. For a practice purchase we want an attorney that has competence in tax and contract work. ASK PROSPECTIVE ATTORNEYS WHAT AREA OF THE LAW THEY PREFER—don't tell them what you need and see if that "just happens" to be their specialty.

Lawyers can also be helpful in giving you an unbiased description of your exact business situation. If nothing else good can be said for this beleaguered profession, they do possess the ability to be brutally frank. They can also negotiate with the seller or seller's attorney on your behalf. (It's often tough for an inexperienced dentist to defend yourself adequately in the confrontational situation of buying an office with some very big money on the table.) They can also draft or modify the seller's contract to protect your interests (read butt!).

I would suggest you phone a number of attorneys and speak with them briefly about your immediate concerns. Have a clear idea of the questions you wish to ask, as these are busy professionals, and record each one's answers. Select a couple of finalists from this list and set up appointments to meet with each personally and discuss your situation. Employ the one you feel most positive about. The time, effort and expense involved in buying a practice makes such diligence worth the trouble. Much as I hate to be the bearer of sad tidings, you will need a skilled attorney fairly often in the course of your career.

In Keokuk there would most likely be no charge for an attorney's office or phone consultation. The local lawyers are sharp enough to consider you a valuable prospective client. When you make the appointment, I would ask the receptionist what charge for a brief office visit is customary. You may find out right away that you aren't able to afford the attorney of your choice at this point in your career.

An associate agreement, again according to the ADA, should cost between $750 to $1,500 to be drafted (mine was $500). A sale contract runs about $2,000.

## Accountant

During a sale YOUR accountant can help project office cash flow and assist you in preparing financial statements for the bank. I make an effort to follow the ever-changing tax codes . . . a significant effort. I can't do it. The morass of tax law is too complex for me to clearly comprehend at a level from which every successful business person must function. You simply must have professional help.

A good accountant is a vital asset to any business, and will prove essential to you throughout your career. You should spend many more hours and dollars dealing with accountants than attorneys, unless you develop an affinity for lawsuits, or they for you. Interview accounting candidates to see who you are comfortable with, then also get a list of PROFESSIONAL CLIENTS OF THEIRS (not some retired families, or people near the poverty level) AND CHECK THE REFERENCES. Good advice from your accountant can help a great deal over the course of a career. Bad advice can destroy you with unnecessary taxes, and the tax effects on an office sale are very significant.

I am going to blithely ignore the tax ramification of a practice sale. The ADA booklet has some good information on the subject, but the tax codes change nationally about every three years. State and local taxes also have an effect. I'm afraid any attempt I make to guide you concerning this complex but critical subject may inadvertently mislead you. Your accountant should be of more value to you with taxes than most attorneys, and will also usually prove a much less expensive source of information.

## Practice Broker

It seems many appraisers are glad to not only value but sell the office, too. Can you see the conflict of interests that exists? For a sale the broker will receive 8 to 12% of the office price. (For my office that's roughly $40,000, created by my blood, sweat and years.) The higher the value the appraiser places on the office, the greater the broker's commission! (In Iowa we call that hiring a fox to guard the chickens.)

To "earn" this amount they search out buyers, screen them to avoid people who have no way to afford the purchase, negotiate a deal and help the buyer arrange financing. Brokers advertise in the ADA, state and city dental journals. Your state and local dental societies may also be able to help you locate these individuals.

Once again, (do you sense a trend in the selection of professional assistance?) interview several, determine which you feel comfortable with and then check references before making this important choice.

Let me re-emphasize that this review of the office practice valuation system is skeletal in nature. Many entire books have been written on the subject. I hope I've touched on the main points in a clear manner that all of you can—with some struggle—come to understand, but you must have professional help during the purchase of an office. Reading the ADA booklet we've repeatedly discussed is also minimal preparation to be competent concerning this complex subject. Consider this need an annoying but **absolutely essential** part of the cost of doing business. A poorly structured deal may take years from which to recover.

Now let's examine the whys and wherefores of starting an office from scratch.

## Chapter Ten

# Flying Solo

We have reached the final segment of our tripartite practice venue choices. After considering joining a group and buying an existing practice, we'll now look full upon a sight that has caused many a strong soul to pale: Beginning an office on your own.

As I've related, this was my own path of choice, but 1974 was a different and distant era. Still a time when dentists, at least in some locations, were in great demand. Opening your own office was a lot more common then, with groups still accounting for but a small percentage of total dental offices. Also recall that I had the advantage of two excellent years of clinical experience in the U.S. Army plus two summers as an extern with Dr. David Shaw—a wonderfully skilled and patient mentor. But I believe more than any other factor, it was my own bullheaded and independent nature that led me to strike out on my own.

Jo and I considered all three practice modes—visiting groups, offices for sale and solo opportunities. (I didn't have this book to help me clarify my thoughts.) Yet, when every office on our list had been evaluated, our final three choices were all solo opportunities. I believe my value clarification occurred during the course of our weeks of journeying to the varied office opportunities we had identified, without my conscious awareness. (Jo suggests that another factor could be that no dentist would put up with me. That's a different slant on the issue.)

What do I feel are the personal attributes that make one suited for solo practice? (Other than my own aforementioned inherent obnoxiousness.)

### 1. Clinical Excellence (Or competence at least)

The solo dentist must have, at minimum, a good basic command of every dental specialty. My two years in the military and six months with Dr. Shaw, where I worked most diligently (honest!) were essential to my being able to successfully begin a practice on my own—but then I'm sort of slow.

Some of you may leave school with the necessary abilities to immediately open a solo practice, but as an old dental school clinical instructor, allow me to tell you that these gifted folks are few and far between. Military service, a residency or group practice experience may be required for most before they possess the clinical excellence required to attempt to establish their own practice.

You must be relatively skilled at ALL the sub-specialties before becoming sequestered in your own little office. While it's not impossible to learn technique on your own, it's sure a lot harder than when someone who already possesses the skills is available to guide you.

### 2. Acute Business Senses

If you can fix teeth like a son of a gun, but not figure out how to make a profit doing it, you'll soon be broke. There are many resources out there to help you. My own first two books leap quickly to mind, but you must possess the **interest and ability in business matters** to continue to confront the constantly changing world of commerce. (And in every season you'll be faced with new challenges, as well as opportunities.)

### 3. Clear Values

I can't possibly be redundant here, as no other attribute is so critical, or so overlooked, on the road to success and joy. Only those with clearly thought-out values are able to take the decisive action required daily to run their own office. As a leader, you must create a vision of your office, and reinforce this vision constantly. You must be able to deal with conflict in an effective and constructive way. Solo practice is not an ideal situation for the timid and/or insecure—or at least for those who choose to remain that way.

### 4. High Energy

The fuel needed to drive a successful solo practice is a burning desire to be your best. Running your own office—at least doing it well—is not possible if you plan to work a 40-hour week. You must become expert on every clinical, management and financial matter. Excuse the hyperbole, but solo practice is a hero's quest, where the challenges never cease—and simply showing up for work isn't enough.

### 5. Reading this Book

Those who have studied this text carefully have already set themselves apart from the great majority of dental practitioners. You had to search out this resource, order and pay for it, and then devote hours to studying the text and following up on the advice you have been given. (Is "blessed with" too strong?)

True, reading this book is but one small example, but it personifies the type of behavior required to successfully manage your own dental office.

## Advantages of a Solo Practice

### 1. Income

If done well, solo practice offers a much greater financial reward than is available from group practice employment. This is consistent with the risk-reward investment philosophy we have discussed. The increased risk of failure in any venture must be countered by the promise of a greater reward for success. To deal with the multiple migraines of solo private practice and not get well paid for the effort is a form of insanity difficult for me to comprehend.

## 2. Freedom

This is the sticking point for many. Dentistry is still one of the few remaining bastions of the fiercely independent business person. Each decade we see other small businesses disappear—swallowed whole by industrial behemoths. The family grocery stores of my youth and more recently the independent practices of pharmacies and optometrists have all but vanished. As I write, medicine and dentistry are drifting ever closer to outside ownership and/or control. But our time of independence isn't quite over yet.

There is a thrill for many of us at being master of our ship—guardian of our own destiny. If this concept concerns you more than it thrills you, seek a group.

## 3. Problem Solving

There exists, for some hardy souls at least, a satisfaction in meeting problems face to face and defeating them. Do you find confronting real difficulties exciting? You won't lack for them in private practice! (The author is compelled by honesty to admit that 20-plus years of solving, often the same problems, has diluted some of the joy from the process for him personally.)

## 4. Control

You are able to create an environment where the only limits are your own abilities, energy and imagination. Some of us could ask for little more.

Many of you have heard doom and gloom predictions concerning our profession, but dentists are unquestionably among the most wealthy 1% of people that have existed in the history of the world! (And yet we whine.) Our profession is liberally sprinkled with self-made millionaires. This book can help launch you on a similar course, if that is an accomplishment you desire.

# Disadvantages to Solo Practice

## 1. Pressure

In a solo practice the owner-doctor is solely responsible for solving every type of problem, and the bombardment never ceases. Staff, patients, government interference, taxes, insurance, legal conundrums—and if you're successful, money management and investing—are merely some of the pressures you'll be forced to perpetually contend with. There is no end!

### 2. You must be the boss

In a solo office, there is nobody else who will accept the infamous buck. There may be staff meetings where the vote is 10 to 1 for, but the single vote is yours and it's nay. Against carries! Such independent action has yet to endear me to my co-workers, but the office bears my name. I spent the eight years of advanced education and many thousands of dollars creating the practice and I'm **also the one who will be sued.** In short, it is my office and thus it's my sole responsibility to do what I feel best—despite any and all advice I may receive to the contrary. True, I can delegate tasks to staff members, but I can never abandon my personal responsibility to see that each assignment is properly completed.

### 3. You're always on call

Twenty-four hours a day, seven days a week patients can find you when dental disasters strike. No emergency room coverage for dentists, at least where I live. Thank God Dr. Long is here to share these obligations with me now, but for 11 years it was my burden to shoulder alone.

### 4. Potential for financial ruin

Just as you have the potential for great gain, an error on your part can lead to ruin. A mistake on a third-party plan contract can prove to be a disaster. Malpractice suit or suits, tax errors, POOR INVESTMENTS—each can nullify all of your efforts.

### 5. Lack of professional companionship and support

Truly, nobody knows the troubles I've seen, except another dentist. Having the wisdom and skill of a fellow doctor available in your office is great, but so is the moral support and compassion when all is not well.

## 6. Competitive disadvantages with groups

We've discussed before how marketing and the utilization of expensive equipment can be performed much more efficiently in a group setting. If you have no experience in practice this may not seem a major factor, but allow me to assure you that it is. Panorex, intra-oral cameras, and other large-ticket items are challenging for solo doctors to finance and afford.

I'm sure you've realized that a great deal of the information needed to begin a solo practice you already possess. The changes required for this venue will be more of emphasis, rather than new content.

As we've stated, clear values and personal vision are even more imperative for those committed to forming a solo office. When merging with an existing practice you must learn the culture of the group and develop your own vision within the confines of this joint culture of which you have elected to become a member.

When you purchase an office, systems and people trained to implement them are already in place. Certainly you can and should change them in a manner consistent with your own beliefs, but the adjustments should take place slowly and gradually so the effects won't be too disruptive.

Beginning a solo office means starting with a blank page. A great opportunity to create, but EVERYTHING (what color office stationery do you choose and on what grade paper?) must be defined by you. Only a clear and consistent vision can guide you through the morass of necessary decisions to create a comprehensive office plan that gives life to your dream, rather than birthing a quivering and confused mass of unrelated choices.

After you have created a clear mental image of the office you will soon have, there follows a search for a community that is consistent with the lifestyle ingredients you and your spouse have identified as important. For a solo office, this quest will exactly follow the basic guidelines we dealt with previously.

**The search to identify practice opportunities will be your greatest challenge.** Dental schools, state and local dental societies may have letters on file from communities searching for a dentist. But there are no want ads or broker interests for offices that don't exist. The assistance of dental supply representatives will prove most critical.

Supply companies are listed in the Yellow Pages and their employees routinely visit every dental school. The staff members of every dental office in the areas in which you have an interest can provide you with the name and number of each dental supply representative that regularly calls on their office. You must cultivate a relationship with **every** representative who calls on the communities you have an interest in—the more sources you have searching, the more opportunities will be identified. Also, it's reassuring—maybe downright exciting—to have three independent representatives all mention the same location. These folks won't be hard to find or to work with, as they wish to help you. If they are instrumental in helping you locate a suitable property and establish an office, they will be rewarded well before heaven for their efforts—by many years of your business.

Recall that dental supply representatives are aware of the towns that are growing and where new industry is locating. They know the communities where most of the doctors are nearing retirement or where every office is always busy when they visit. They may even be aware of suitable office space that is available.

Compare the opportunities they discuss with the ideal living conditions you desire for the community you will call home. Then call chamber of commerce offices and search the library for data on these possible locations.

A quick start to your business is more critical when beginning on your own, as no patients await you. ***SELECTING THE RIGHT BUSINESS OPPORTUNITY IS ESSENTIAL.*** Productive efforts in office location selection will be rewarded with a lifetime of success. The cost of failure will be measured in wasted years. You still want to find a town that is consistent with your desires for living the life of your dreams, but the area's need for a dentist must now be very high on—if not atop—your list of factors to consider.

Once you have identified some likely locations, call ahead and speak to area bankers, realtors and the local dentists. These sources may refer you to additional individuals who can help in your quest for information.

The dentists you contact may not be glad you called. Today, few welcome more competition—but call you must. This is just one small example of the need to go outside your comfort zone to achieve success that private practice demands. I would again (always) have a prepared set of questions to ask each person you contact. Topics such as those we've been discussing about the local economy and area business as well as the housing market are appropriate for realtors.

The bankers' interest in financing a new dental practice is among the major concerns about which you'll wish to enquire. They are also an excellent resource of information concerning the local economy. Banks' willingness to loan to dentists varies greatly by area of the country as well as during the various financial cycles our economy passes through. Don't spend days working on a practice, only to finally discover it is impossible to get financial assistance in this area. Banks vary greatly in their tendencies to work with professionals, and if the institutions in one community aren't receptive to your needs, it doesn't mean banks in another location won't be.

As for your conversations with dentists, you'll wish to befriend them and gather what information you can. These people may become your colleagues, hopefully even good friends. Perhaps—if your call goes well—you can arrange to visit their offices later and meet with them personally? Among the many queries you may wish to express, the two key questions are:

1. Is your office as busy as you wish it to be?
2. What type of business opportunity for another dentist do you believe exists in your community?

No other source can possibly answer these vital questions as accurately as the area dentists.

You will visit with some dentists who are gracious and friendly. I'm afraid a few may do all they can to discourage you. Remember, NO ONE BIT OF INFORMATION, BE IT POSITIVE OR NEGATIVE, IS ENOUGH TO SINGLEHANDEDLY LEAD TO A DECISION. The answers the area dentists give you, and the tone of their discourse, are just single pieces—albeit important ones—of the overall practice location puzzle.

Let's assume you and your spouse have done your homework. You've identified the characteristics of the community of your dreams and you personally have created a vision for the office you desire, be it a cottage or palace. You've screened every possible practice site you've been able to identify. After studying information about the potential locations, as well as many phone conversations with local community leaders and area dentists, you have narrowed your choices to a workable few. It's finally time for a road trip!

Your visit to the community will be exactly as we previously discussed. You must schedule appointments in advance to meet with realtors—hopefully several—to see what office and home accommodations are available. Jo and I used to separate in the morning, she looking for living quarters (of course we discussed in detail what we desired, "cheap" being the predominant feature) while I looked at potential office space. We'd meet for lunch, compare notes, then together revisit the home and office locations we felt had promise. Remember to dedicate a spiral notebook to this enterprise and take careful notes on everything.

You'll also want to meet with local bank officers, preferably one from each area bank and savings and loan, to glean further information about the local economy and to find out exactly how willing they are to be of assistance to you with your capital needs. We'll carefully discuss the critical subject of how to approach financing a dental office in the following chapter.

I'll leave living accommodations to the purview of you and your good spouse. Allow me to discuss identification of potential office locations. **The first step is to create an office in your mind.** How many operatories will you equip and how many total would you like to have potentially available? (How large an office and how intensely you choose to work are the key questions to be answered here.)

What will the design and decor look like—pleasantly middle-class or upscale? The type of dentistry you prefer defines in great part the area within the community in which you will ideally be located. If you visualize a family dental practice, your ideal location might be in an area where new family homes are being constructed, possibly near a school.

This would be markedly different from a removable prosthodontist's or full mouth reconstruction dentist's choice. (Hint: Think mansions!) You wish to locate your office near the TYPE of client you wish to serve. All this is part of your vision.

There are several books on office design, all available on loan from the ADA library. (Phone 800-621-8099.) There are books available which contain hundreds of office blueprints that even I can understand. These resources will prove invaluable in the creation of your office vision.

Most major dental supply houses also have staff trained and experienced in office design and will usually assist you on a pro bono basis (free!). Of course, the final design will have to be tailored to fit the available space—few of us start out constructing our own building, wonderful as that would be. But the general office concept must be clearly in mind before you can accurately evaluate existing locations.

What do I think you should look for? MY PERSONAL OPINION is that you should seek a balance as regards size. Not too small to restrict your future growth, yet not so large that you can't afford it. This probably describes a space of about 1,000 square feet, give or take 200. The give or take will vary by your concept of an office—big and busy or smaller and more calm. It will vary by your personal finances, as well as the characteristics of the building you choose and the subsequent level of rent. **Mostly it will vary by your honest self-evaluation and confidence.** If you believe in yourself—your ability and drive to achieve—and feel the great effort you have put forth to find an excellent location has been successful, you can engage more space in a larger, costlier building.

I would design an office with room for three operatories and would immediately equip two, while having a third wired and plumbed, ready to go in service the moment I need it. (It is both much cheaper and more convenient to have the needed wiring and plumbing completed during the leasehold improvement stage than to hire contractors to come back and do the job at the time you are ready to actually add the additional room.)

I would have a lab, private office and reception area. I would advise you to go with a larger than usually suggested business office. This is the nerve center of the practice and, as you get busy, business needs will quickly expand to fill the available space.

When I enlarged my office I allowed the business center over 350 square feet. When the office was completed I looked at this mostly empty space and thought it would never be used. Today it is crammed and we're searching for storage space to rent for the overflow. *If you accept a space unable to accommodate the minimum I have just described, you'll be severely limiting your ability to succeed and grow.*

Continuing my personal opinions, I'd initially hire two employees, one receptionist and a chairside. We'll have two full chapters devoted to staff hiring and team building. The proper staff will make or break you. Working on the team building ideas we'll discuss is essential, and when your office is just beginning, you should have plenty of time to devote to this vital task.

In both staffing and creating a physical plant, plan for success. Don't spend beyond your means, but don't allow a limited office design and staff capability to create a situation where you can't grow. These two factors are the most critical concerns as regards your potential for success next to the ability, effort and desire of the doctor.

## Lease

Let's assume you've examined a community and found some suitable potential office locations. The next step is negotiating a lease. I am NOT an expert here. I have owned the space I practice in for many years. I did own and manage two rental properties for about 10 years. (What a nightmare that investment was. It only seemed like eternity!) I will gladly pass on what information I do possess about leases.

You must understand that leases are very negotiable. If the area you're interested in has several potential office locations available, YOU'RE IN THE DRIVER'S SEAT. If you've only identified one suitable spot, you have less leverage, but remember the owner wants the space rented as badly as you wish to secure it.

There are many ways in which the lease negotiations can be handled. Sometimes up to three months of free rent will be granted to a starting business. You may be able to get the landlord to build the office to your design, or at least remodel, at his or her own expense in exchange for a higher rent or longer lease. (Much more on this concept later.)

You need to keep as much flexibility as possible in the leasing arrangement, as it's impossible to predict how long it will be before you'll outgrow this space. Does the lease allow you to sublet to another renter if you need to move on? (Subletting means you are allowed to rent to another tenant of your choosing, but you personally remain committed to fulfilling all the terms of the lease with your original landlord.)

There are many variables to explore, depending on the needs of both you and the landlord. For instance, if the building owner is in acute financial distress, they can't offer the first few months rent-free. If they have a tax problem the year you move in, they may be pleased to delay rent payments, and thus defer their income into the following year. You could possibly receive lower monthly rent for a longer lease commitment. Or a lower first-year rent for a higher rate in following years. Work to get the best deal possible. It's wise to have your attorney review the actual lease, but these documents are usually pretty standard and there may not be too much your attorney can do to alter the contract provisions.

You must begin to study the lease early in the evaluation process, to be sure you do indeed have a possible office location available in the community. However, don't sign a lease—a binding legal obligation—until you are absolutely certain this is THE location for your first office. You might ask the local dentists what they consider to be a reasonable rent for the area where you will be working. Typical rent for a high-rise office space in San Francisco is a bit more than my space in Keokuk would command.

## Equipment and Supplies

Any dental supply company will be delighted to give you a checklist of all possible supplies and equipment you will need to open your office. You solo candidates must be in contact with these companies anyway, so I won't waste the paper reproducing the list here. I do have a few observations I believe will prove helpful.

Attending major dental meetings—like the largest of them all, the Midwinter in Chicago, or the annual ADA meeting—will allow you to see and compare equipment carefully, virtually side by side. Dealers almost always have fairly generous specials and discounted prices at these meetings, so it is possible that you can learn a great deal about equipment at the meeting and pay for your trip expense with your savings from purchases made there.

Smaller dental meetings, even state ones, usually don't have the same number of exhibitors in attendance. There may be only the big-name, and thus often higher-priced, equipment companies represented.

When you are purchasing an entire office, supply houses should be willing to offer substantial discounts. You may be able to get as much as 20% off the list price, but such a discount won't be volunteered. You must make an offer. Assume your total for some major equipment came to $16,000. Offer the dealer 20% less—$12,800. If you get bids from several supply houses, one will probably accept the offer. Don't hesitate to re-approach a dealer with a lower competitive bid and give him an opportunity to beat the estimate. Continue this process until the lowest possible estimate is obtained.

(Feels good to think of all the thousands of dollars I've saved my readers with this one paragraph. I was a dentist ten years before it occurred to me to offer a bid on equipment, and I was stunned when they quickly accepted!)

A critical item will be the dental chairs and units you select. It has been my PERSONAL EXPERIENCE that with dental chairs and units you often don't get what you pay for. I have had more success with some of the less expensive models than with the "brand names" that sold for double their price. Be sure to sit in each chair personally, as the difference in comfort from model to model is surprisingly great.

The compressor and vacuum systems are the heart and lungs of your office. When either of them fails, the office is closed. I'd buy the best quality possible here.

It really pays to shop for dental materials and supplies. The cost of equipping and furnishing an office will most likely exceed what you spend furnishing your home! Take your time and look around. There are bargains available. I always ask the service people which models they feel hold up best and which are easiest for them to repair (everything breaks eventually). I can't judge by looking which chair represents the best value, and if you ask fellow dentists, they can only provide information about the few models they have personally purchased. The people who actually install and repair equipment are by far the most knowledgeable and unbiased source of information available. Be clear, I refer to the service representatives, not your friendly supply and equipment salesman.

Consider your vision again. As pertains to dental materials, there seems to be no substitute for the best. Good technique can't compensate for a ineffective lab or poor-quality supplies.

I use four different laboratories, a separate one for each type of lab work I require. I have never found a lab capable of producing consistent quality for every type of dental procedure in which I needed their assistance. I have painstakingly identified these labs over the years by trial and error (and not a few remakes!). I've never found a cheap lab that did good work, and I've tried a few. You will pay for an excellent lab and your fees must reflect this expense. There is an old dental saying that it's a lot easier to explain the bill than excuse a clinical failure. The saying is true. I hope your office vision will include your performing only the quality of care for every patient you treat that you'd wish your loved ones to receive.

The least expensive and most efficient way we have found to order supplies, once you have identified the precise materials you desire, is from a company called THE PROFIT FINDER. (Phone 800-624-7467.) They use a proprietary computer software to find the lowest available price for the specific brand name products you request. It's impossible to review every catalog and check each sale for the lowest price for gloves at the moment you need them, but that's what these folks do for a living. Call them for complete information. I'm sorry to say I don't get a kickback if you decide to use them.

Choosing which materials work the best is a constant challenge in our ever-changing industry. The best source of data ON THE FACE OF THE EARTH is the *Clinical Research Associates Newsletter*. This fine and inexpensive source of unbiased information is published by Dr. Gordon J. Christensen, Ph.D., D.D.S.—arguably America's preeminent dentist. They offer video courses, on-the-site training and lectures nationwide. I highly recommend their newsletter and you can reach these nice people at 801-226-2121. (They don't pay me either.)

A surprisingly large expense for your new office will be floor- and wall-covering. I've redone my office many times and let me tell you as forcefully as I can ***THAT IT PAYS TO GO WITH QUALITY HERE!*** A good industrial carpet will hold up beautifully until you're sick of looking at it. I would use all carpet, if that is still an issue. In the "old days" linoleum was often recommended for floor-covering in the operatories. The new pre-measured amalgam mixes eliminate mercury spills and carpet is a much nicer, quieter surface. It even lasts and looks better much longer.

## Summary

I know this has been a lot of information, and yet not nearly enough. We've still far to go, with securing financing and attracting patients next on our agenda. Let's now concisely review the key points we've discussed to date. You'd never guess what's first.

1. Everything must begin with your creation of a home community and office vision. (Surprised?) You must smell your office (scented candles and popcorn, not formalin), see the soft incandescent light in the reception room. (People WAIT in waiting rooms. Ours is there to receive them.)

   My reception area is as much like a living room as possible, with a play area for kids and a picture of my family on the wall. I like the parents that wait anxiously for their kids to know I have children too.

2. Search out possible locations in communities that meet your guidelines. The dental supply people will be your key resource. Overturn every stone in your search for opportunities, but work especially hard with the dental supply representatives. Remember, choosing this location will be one of the biggest decisions of your life!

3. Interview realtors, bankers and area dentists by phone.
   How is the local economy?
   Are the bankers willing, even eager to work with you?
   Are there potential office spaces available?
   How do you feel about the aggregate response of the local dentists? Have they been encouraging about the prospects of your new office?

4. Look over the community in general. Meet with the bankers in person. Have the realtors guide your search for office space and housing. AT THIS POINT, DETERMINE IF FINANCING

IS AVAILABLE AND DOES A POTENTIAL OFFICE SPACE EXIST? If not, it's time to repeat the above-listed process in another location.

5. If you have identified a space that will allow creation of your office vision, begin to work with the landlord on a lease agreement. Remember all we've discussed about negotiations here.
6. It's now time to begin to research and order the equipment and supplies you'll need to select well in advance. You don't want to sit for months waiting for the office to be ready. Remember, you're broke, and as a doctor, probably can't get your old job back at McDonald's.

   A trip to a major dental meeting—and of course you can't afford it—will pay real dividends in your being able to directly compare equipment and save money purchasing the meeting price specials. Don't forget to place a bid for the equipment, not just pay full price.
7. Staff hiring and training. There are two full chapters upcoming on this subject, but the staff has to be selected and trained before you open the office doors. It takes me TWO MONTHS to hire and minimally train staff.
8. The moment you signed a lease, begin working on the design for this space. The books you've been reading and the work you've done with the supply houses have prepared you to do this job yourself. If you are building an office from the ground up, you should have an architect's assistance, but if you put your mind to it, I believe all of you can successfully design an office within an existing space. It will take many hours, so be prepared and start early.
9. You'll need to find contractors to do the office construction, and again, get BIDS from several. Usually a general contractor will have the electricians and plumbers available for you (lots of plumbing in a dental office!) and their special costs will be a part of the total bid. It can take *two months* to find the contractors, select a bid, and have them ready to *begin* the cre-

ation of your vision. If the area you choose to locate in is experiencing a lot of building, the wait could be much longer.

10. Here's a list of the simple, yet essential tasks remaining:

    a) Be sure you have a state license! Contact the state board for information.

    b) Obtain a federal and state narcotics license. Contact:
       Drug Enforcement Administration
       U.S. Department of Justice
       Washington, D.C. 20537

    c) You must have a federal employer I.D. number. Your accountant can obtain it, or you can contact the Internal Revenue Service in your district (they're in the phone book) and ask for form SS-4.

    d) Secure a state employer I.D. from your accountant or contact the state department of revenue.

    e) Contact your local hospital for staff privileges. Being on staff will at least usually reduce your family's hospital bills if any of you ever require treatment (thanks to customary staff discounts), even if you never treat a patient in the hospital.

    f) TELEPHONE NUMBER. Contact the phone company the DAY you sign the lease. The phone book only comes out once a year, and it can be a long wait to get your office number listed. Try to obtain a number that is easy for people to remember. For example, our office number is 8811.

Let's now enter the intimidating world of finance. We can't create an office if we can't secure the money to begin one, and obtaining financial assistance can be a very real and serious problem.

## Chapter Eleven

# Creating the Plane

It behooves us little to fantasize about flying solo if we have no plane. In our case the necessary aircraft is a fully equipped dental office from which we may perform our barrel rolls or aerial acrobatics of choice. But airplanes and dental offices are expensive. You are a new graduate, or close to it, with your only financial achievement worthy of note being DEBT! How can we possibly hope to buy our own most essential airplane? Will we be forced by these circumstances to forever be mere copilots in another's craft?

Many of you reading these words have school debts in the $40,000 to $80,000 range. Your assets consist of worn clothing and a ten-year-old car. When I first seriously considered locating in Keokuk, I made appointments with the highest officer I was allowed to see in each community bank. I received interest and offers of help from all three of the local institutions. But I had savings (albeit a modest $10,000) and no appreciable school debt. Also, my times were the 1970's. The world in general, and banks in particular, have changed a great deal since my salad days.

We'll discuss bank loans—the old-fashioned way of financing. But for many of you this simply won't be an option. Fortunately we have the wisdom of Dr. Howard Farran to rely upon. Howard is a 1990's guy. He finished dental school with a self-proclaimed $86,000 of debt and was producing over $1,000,000 within three years in an office he started from scratch! (Such an accomplishment may seem unattainable, but as my daddy says, if it's already been done, chances are it's possible.)

Howard lectures to many dental groups all over our great land. He publishes a monthly newsletter, entitled *The Farran Report*, and has an excellent book available called *The Business of Dentistry*. You may reach Howard by calling 602-598-9757. Allow me to say that Howard is revolutionary in his thinking. (Hell, Howard is a revolution!) What follows is his description of how a new graduate with no money can start the solo office of your dreams.

You'll all recognize that the following information wasn't drawn from my experience, and I try to limit the pathways I describe, as much as possible, to my actual accomplishments. (Who said this may be a short book?) But Howard is such a unique resource that I present his thoughts to you with no reservations. To do less would be depriving my readers of information of great value.

The key to capitalism—the economic system so near and dear to the hearts of most Americans—is the establishment of a mechanism which allows the ready availability of capital or money. It is to make money attainable and to stimulate economic growth that our federal treasury and banking institutions were developed. The lack of a system that allows money to flow to viable economic concerns is what dooms the Third World countries to unending poverty.

I hope every reader is aware of my aversion to debt. That will never change. But there is a significant difference between using other people's money (OPM) to create a business, and entering the shadowy halls of debt to purchase objects—toys—that you haven't as yet earned the right to possess.

The high debt of today's graduates may make a less radical start-up plan than Howard details—such as working as an associate and saving—next to impossible to accomplish. The double whammy of student loan payments and taxes on your income (and student loan interest is no longer—since 1986—a tax-deductible item) may mean many years of living poorly and struggling to get out of debt before even considering beginning to save for an office of your own.

The aggressive path we are about to disclose hinges on piling additional debt on top of existing loans. In any business venture, greater debt burden means an increased chance of financial failure. If this is the path you choose to follow, success hinges on your ability to establish an early and solid cash flow. To achieve this you must have:

1. Found an excellent location where a dentist is indeed needed—a topic we have dealt with at length—but due to the economic pressures of additional debt, this is now imperative to our practice's survival.
2. Be able to create a large flow of patients in a short period of time. This takes place through marketing your practice, a matter we will attend to in this chapter.
3. Be astutely and acutely aware of the reality that you are entering the ***BUSINESS OF DENTISTRY***. High debt levels mated with a lack of essential business awareness can produce but one offspring . . . BANKRUPTCY.

Let's begin by adding the final bit of information on office location. Here we deal with micro-location, i.e., the ideal location within the community of your choice. The key is to find a spot that is highly visible—where many people will view your office as they pass by each day. A location on a heavily traveled street is excellent. Also, grocery stores are where moms—the people who make the overwhelming majority of dental appointments—spend a great deal of their time. Your office being located near a prominent grocery assures high visibility.

Assume we've identified a possible office location on a major road, within sight of the town's largest and most busy grocery store, and 1,000 square feet of space is available immediately!

But we still have no plane (office) and no money with which to purchase one. How can this bare space become the office we have envisioned in our dreams?

Allow me to use (actually, steal from Howard) some rough, but fairly accurate figures to illustrate our points. Let's assume you've determined the investment cost to turn this open space into a dental office—with all the special plumbing and wiring, and a quality, serviceable but not lavish interior—to be $40 per square foot. For our 1,000 feet this expense would amount to a total of $40,000. The cost of improving a typical non-dental space is approximately $10 per foot—an expense which the landlord will expect to pay. This leaves us with a net $30,000 shortfall.

Before talking to the landlord, call the Board of Dental Examiners in your state and ask them how many dental licenses have been revoked in the last five years. You'll find the number most likely to be in single digits. Share this information with your prospective landlord to illustrate that a dental office is an excellent business risk. You're much less likely to go broke in this space, and default on the lease, than some little shop or restaurant. We in the profession know this to be the case and must be certain the landlord understands the stability and desirability of a dentist as a tenant.

Let's assume you will sign a standard five-year lease. We will need $30,000 in total, or $6,000 per year to finish our space in the manner we desire. This calculates out to $6 per square foot annually. The landlord should agree to perform the leasehold improvements to your specifications in exchange for a $6 per foot increase in rent that will return the $30,000 over the five year term of the lease. In essence, you use higher rent payments to finance your office construction expenses.

We have now established an ideal location and an office is being built on the spot, to our precise specifications. The next step is to equip our space—install the engine in our plane.

Go to the major dental supply companies in your area, such as Patterson. Carefully select good equipment, but tell them the limits of your budget. You can completely furnish your office with high-quality new equipment, but avoid the most expensive brand-name items. The total investment required to equip a two-operatory office in the above described manner will be around $30,000. Get initial bids from every supply house, then approach each with the competing bids. Continue to give each company a chance to match the ever-dropping bids of their competitors. Keep working the numbers and discuss options until they are sick of you and you of them. You may go through several declarations of "this is our final price" on your way down, but keep discussing cost with each bidder until you are sure no more downside is possible in their estimate. Then accept the lowest bid.

But you have no money? THE DENTAL SUPPLY COMPANY WILL LEASE THE EQUIPMENT TO YOU. This is a very standard arrangement within our profession, much as automobile manufacturers now finance car purchases themselves. If your office fails, they can repossess the equipment, so their risk is not great.

But, how do you live until the cash starts coming in? How do you pay those little bills which demand attention with no money and no source of income? Simply fill out a credit card application, doctor, and you have an instant $5,000 line of credit to tide you over until office cash flow begins. The card you receive will undoubtedly charge you a high rate of interest —possibly 19% or more. Be certain this is the first debt you repay!

Howard suggests one other alternative to opening your office with no money. (He knows TWO ways!) Call the ADA and ask them to give you the names of companies who will sell you a list of dentists 55 years of age or older living in the area you have chosen to make your home.

Contact each doctor and explain you are an eager, engaging and gifted young graduate, willing to purchase an office. However, they must be willing to finance the acquisition for you. Remember, the cost of the office will be higher if they agree to hold the debt personally, due to their greater risk, as we have discussed—but self-financing by the seller of a dental office is common.

Howard and I share a mutual dislike for working with banks and savings and loans. They can be extremely cautious and often slow to make loans and can prove to be frustrating and demeaning to deal with. Yet the time will likely arrive when you will need to secure a loan. I have yet to borrow from a bank, but I studied to prepare myself for such an event should the need arise. Allow me to share some concepts with you.

Dentists have some trouble getting bank-type financing as we are rumored to be poor business people. The basic cause of this perception is the fact that it is usually true! We have virtually no training to prepare us for the world of finance, but we don't have to stay unprepared. (Has not every reader of this book increased his or her awareness of the business of dentistry by quantum amounts already? And isn't that fact sad considering you've each had at least eight years of college education to prepare you to earn a living?)

When just beginning your office, you have no factual financial basis upon which to be awarded a loan. I would approach a bank with my IDEA. This should be in **narrative form**, telling the bank what you wish to use the loan for and IN WHAT MANNER YOU PLAN TO RETURN THEIR MONEY—the bank's main concern.

Let's say you have opened your office and in three months, due to the tremendous inflow of new patients (from the marketing ideas we're about to discuss) you realize you must employ a hygienist. For some reason, you won't go back to the dental company to finance the needed additional equipment—maybe you wish to gain experience dealing with a bank or establish a line of credit to help secure a mortgage on a new house you now estimate you'll be able to afford within the year.

Approach the bank with all the facts available to you. Your production and collection figures for the months your office has been open and new patient flow can best be illustrated by a bar graph. This shows their rapid growth most dramatically. You can project these figures out for the full year and estimate a possible net profit. The bank officers will also wish to see your current debt status, and the schedule you have created (read "made up" after only three months) to explain how and when you expect to pay these financial obligations off.

The narrative will show the **potential income** from the hygienist using the chair. Let's assume your hygienist will begin seeing patients three days a week and you estimate this will total ten patients per day at $50 per visit. The hygienist's salary will be $160 per day and you estimate $40 daily in supply use and miscellaneous costs. Your income flow is thus $1,500 per week ($500 per day times three days). The direct expense of salary and supplies would total $600 per week. This will leave you with an excess cash flow of $900 per week to service the debt on the room and pay any incidental expenses.

The cost of debt service will vary by the amount of the loan, interest rate paid and length of the note. Your accountant can easily help you estimate the precise figures for your situation.

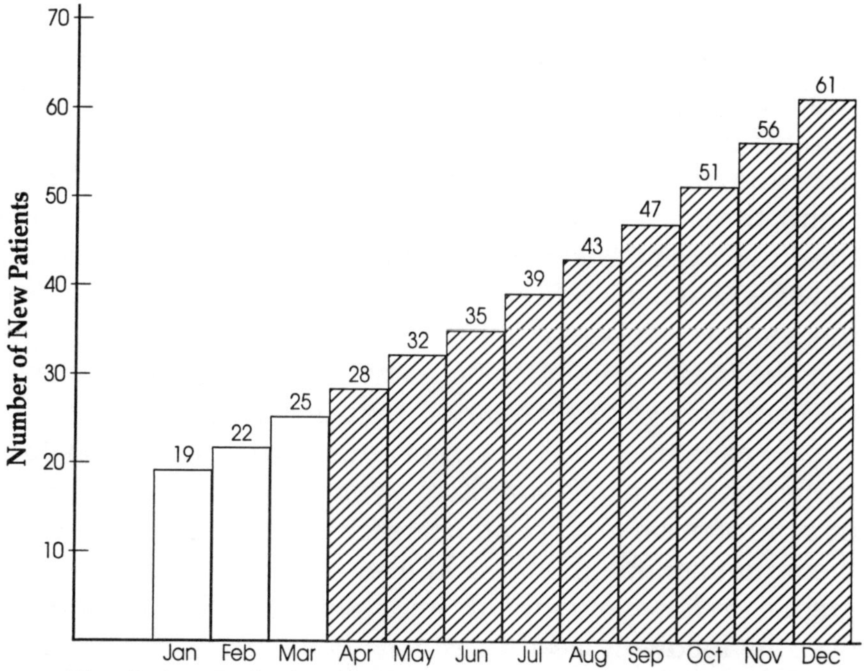


**New Patient Projection (April-December based on 12% growth)**

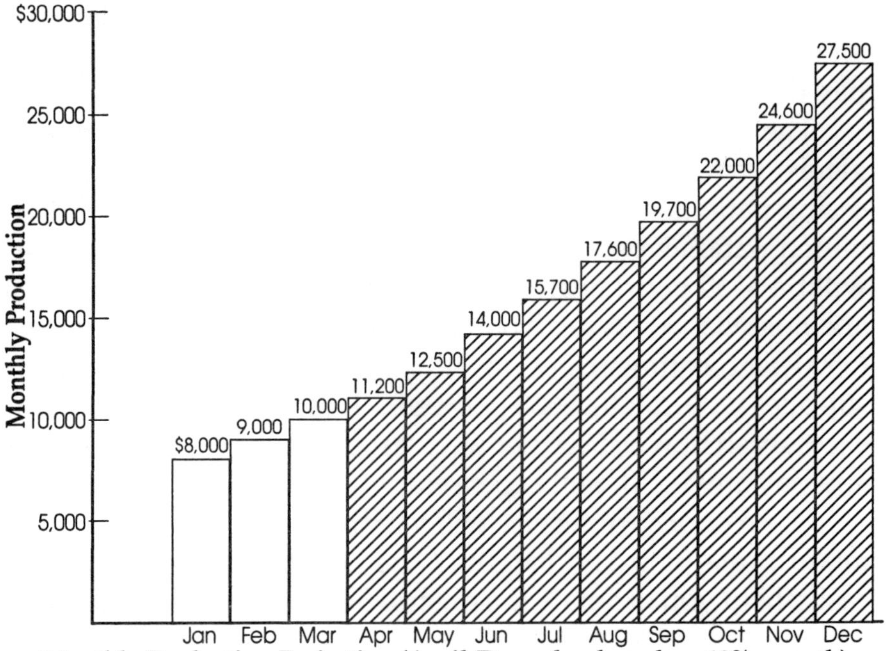


**Monthly Production Projection (April-December based on 12% growth)**

When the information has been prepared in the manner we've described, typed flawlessly on quality paper and presented within an excellent leather portfolio (available from any stationery store, and physical evidence of your willingness to do things right), the bank's okay should be a mere formality. Can you see the difference between this approach and a young dentist sitting down with a bank officer and saying, "I'd like to borrow some money to buy a dental unit?" One exemplifies a business person, the other a child playing grown-up. Successfully repaying the bank note will help establish you as a good credit risk.

We're getting a little ahead of our story, but when you do go to the bank to finance your home, you'll most likely have a year or more of positive office numbers for them to study. I would list these numbers by month, and again, chart the figures on bar graphs to show your growth, and then extrapolate these trends over the following year to estimate your future income potential. Remember, loans are repaid in the future, so it is into this misty domain that bankers must peer to judge the worthiness of a loan application. How can a banker be expected to project income for our profession as accurately as we can, and why would we wish them to even try?

Be aware in your dealings with banks that their officers have virtually no understanding of our profession. They both want and need us to guide them with such information as our most likely (and most optimistic) income projections and debt repayment schedules.

The specific bank officer you discuss a loan with must take the information you have prepared to a bank loan committee and persuade them to approve the credit application. This officer needs your figures as ammunition in this confrontation to have any chance of the loan being authorized. To even bring the loan request before the committee, the officer must first be personally impressed that you are a serious business person who will be an excellent credit risk and valuable long-term customer.

## Establishing Patient Flow

We shift scenes and find you standing in the center of the very office your vision has created, now become reality. The setting is pleasant, if not opulent. The equipment new. The entire effect exudes confidence and substance. We still need to select and train a team, and we'll deal with that critical issue shortly. Right now we have one overwhelming concern: Where do we find patients?

Creating this vision was an exhilarating experience. But recall that the down-side of leverage—using other people's money to compound our return—is additional risk. We need cash coming in the door, and quickly, if our business is to survive.

In this section I'll revert to describing only the marketing we do in our office. Howard has some great ideas in his book concerning direct mail, newsletters, free services coupons and such. We don't engage in said activities within our office, so I will refer you to Dr. Farran's book if you have interest in this type of aggressive practice enhancement. But first take a look at the marketing an old guy like me still does. It may surprise you.

The first step is to develop **THE** dominant Yellow Pages ad for your area phone book.

I believe our ad to be the most effective in our market, but you'll need to research the area in which your practice is located to create that dominance on your own. Your ad should precisely reflect the clear vision of your office. What are the special things you will bring to the practice of dentistry? Do you enjoy treating kids, have special interest in geriatric care, focus on gentleness and compassion, have expanded hours, reasonable fees, offer cash discounts? Proclaim your painstakingly clarified unique identity in the Yellow Pages.

You can't be all things to all people—offering the greatest of everything for the lowest of fees—at least not and stay in business. But you can focus clearly on the things you do believe in and have your ad reflect this image.

A quality Yellow Pages ad is a major expense, although costs vary a lot by region, so consider yours carefully. Call the phone company to find out the cost for the various types of Yellow Pages advertisements available. Remember, you'll have to live with your choice until next year when a new phone book is published. Don't overfill the ad and make it appear cluttered—our current

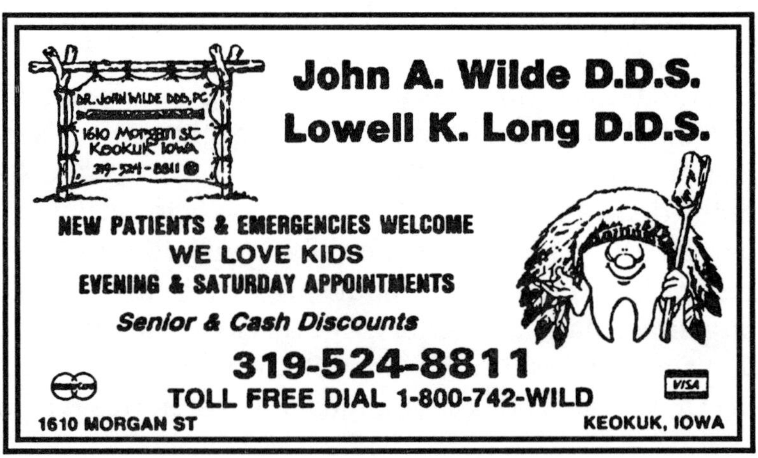

ad is on the brink of committing this error. Blank spaces catch the eye. So do photos or logos, like our silly Indian-hat character.

Yellow Pages ads are half of our office's external marketing campaign. (I believe I can hear Howard laughing at me!) We also offer free dental examinations and bitewing x-rays through our local Welcome Wagon representatives. We are the only area dental office using Welcome Wagon that offers free exams, and we've had a lot of nice people enter our practice because of this value. It doesn't take too many $500 crowns to make up for the $40 lost on the exam. Fearing to lose the exam fee to acquire the patient is a trait of many dentists that has been aptly referred to as "stepping over dollars to save nickels."

You pay a significant fee to join Welcome Wagon and an additional fee for each visit to your potential patients they make. You'll receive a listing monthly of every person they call upon. We phone each one and welcome them to our community (or congratulate them on their wedding, special anniversary or birth of a child—all events Welcome Wagon acknowledges). We ask if they received our complimentary exam and x-ray card and offer to be of service to them in any way we can.

A great number of people have received the card and meant to call, but in the busy circumstances Welcome Wagon acknowledges, haven't gotten around to it yet. They are often delighted to schedule when we call. If you go to the expense of Welcome Wagon, make the follow-up calls religiously. The tone of the call should be low-key and friendly. "We're just calling to say hello and let you know we will be delighted to help you in any way we can." We average about 10 new patients a month from Welcome Wagon alone.

I am also willing to speak in front of any group, anywhere, anytime. I can discuss a dental topic for 20 minutes—about as long a time as prudent before my audience and I both get bored—with no preparation at all (unless you count eight years of schooling and 23 years of experience). I speak to seniors' groups, schools and preschools, service groups and anyone else who asks me, tailoring my topic to the collective interests of the group I'm addressing. It's a method of showing our profession in a positive light and of our office becoming known within the community itself. I even get a free meal once in a while.

The remainder of our marketing consists of activities we perform within the office itself—thus referred to as internal marketing. The obvious key to these efforts is getting people inside the door to positively impress. Direct mailing of coupons for free exams and x-rays—one of Howard's many suggestions—could help to get the ball rolling.

## No Cavity Club

We have the good people at Sematodontics send us a HUGE STUFFED ANIMAL every three months. (Sematodontics can be reached by calling 800-522-0800. They have some great marketing ideas. We buy stickers to give to our child patients from them—something always popular with the little ones—as well as a variety of cards and other practice enhancement ideas.) These big stuffed animals are expensive, in the $60-80 range, but pretty impressive to the kids they tower over. All children we examine who have no decay, or all those who have decay but get it repaired, have their names placed in our No Cavity Club. Once every three months we draw a name and award the animal to the lucky "club member."

Our local newspaper takes a picture of a staff member and the winning (and beaming!) child—firmly clutching the new animal—and publishes it in the paper at no charge to us. They list the names of EVERY KID IN THE NO CAVITY CLUB and some little note I write about how neat it is that these kids are all cavity free. Who doesn't like to see your name in the paper? (Unless you've been arrested.)

## Coloring Contest

Every other month we have a coloring contest. We split the kids into two groups (roughly those who stay within the lines and those outside—I fall forever in the latter) and award a smaller stuffed animal to each winner. My wife, Jo, picks these toys up at Wal-Mart for about $15 each. We decorate the office walls with all the "artwork" generated by our small patients' diligent efforts. Moms, kids and all of us in the office have a great time with the contest. We give a copy of the same picture to each child and the kids can color it in our office if they need to wait for Mom. (The serious ones take the pictures home where they can perform their very best coloring.)

## World-Class Toy Chest

This is Jo's department and she scours the catalogs and exhibits at dental meetings to find the very coolest in toys. She recently bought a whole lot of miniature pacifiers in the form of necklaces. Dumbest thing I ever saw! But we can't keep them in the place—kids love them—even teenagers!

It's really fun to thrill a child with some $.25 toy or three (we're very generous with our toys), as well as the stickers we mentioned. We must have over 100 varieties of toys that fill our treasure chest during any given year. We also have free French fry certificates provided for us by McDonald's at no expense to us that we pass out to every child. Fast-food places can market, and will be delighted to provide some small item you can dispense, knowing it will bring the family into their place of business and create positive feelings for their company.

## Seniors Smile Month

We pick one month a year and celebrate our senior patients. We take a photo of each senior we see in the office and hang their pictures on one of our many bulletin boards. Then at month's end we select one picture at random and send the lucky winner to dinner for two at a local restaurant as our treat. The total cost for this gala event is usually about $40.

Guess what? The paper publishes a photo of the winner and lists all the contestants, along with some words penned by yours truly about the importance of good oral health throughout a lifetime, but especially in our golden years.

## Preschool Visits

During Oral Health Month, we get every preschool we can convince to participate to bring their kids to our office for a visit. They come back to our designated operatory in little bunches and ride in the chair, see the magic straw drink some water and generally have a good time. They all go home with a bag containing a few toys, a French fry certificate, a new tooth-brush and pencil that both just happen to have our office name on them, and—most importantly—a very positive impression of our office as a friendly and fun place.

I think this is a wonderful opportunity to introduce a lot of kids to the pleasant environment of our office specifically and dentistry generally. We eventually see many of these kids as patients, and they can't wait to tell us all they remember about our office from their preschool visit. True, this is marketing, but of all our efforts at making the public aware we exist, this benefits the patients the most and is great fun for all of us.

We have a Sega machine in our reception room our patients can play as our treat, but a new machine costs $3,000. We also have virtual reality glasses for the patients to wear to entertain them and make them more comfortable during dental treatment, but these sell for a hefty $700 each. Both are good marketing tools—kids often bring their friends along to the office to play Sega—but possibly outside the budget of most beginning offices.

Allow me to stress the basic essentials any dental office must consistently perform to succeed, beyond the ideas of marketing we've touched upon.

1. There must be a friendly staff who understand that the patient is always right. The office leader (that's you, doctor) must consistently set this positive tone.

2. The office must see patients ON TIME. In the rare event when this isn't possible, a sincere apology must be offered, along

with a beverage. We'll discuss the need to *time your procedures* in a subsequent chapter, but patients no longer sit quietly, waiting for the doctor to share his or her precious time with them. If the days of tolerant, forgiving patients ever existed, they're now gone.

3. The office must be perpetually neat, clean and professional in appearance. No one refers people to a doctor's office with cobwebs or dust. Your office must always have the appearance of a place patients would be proud to recommend to their friends and family. Our office is professionally cleaned each day. The shiny spotlessness our cleaning lady provides is a true asset to our office.
4. Gentle, predictable and profound anesthetic must be the rule. **Shots can't hurt!** This topic is so essential, we'll devote an entire chapter to it. Today, nobody refers or returns to an office where they have experienced pain.

Each of the above critical topics will be discussed in greater detail as we proceed, but let's start with the most essential topic of them all—forming the team you will surround yourself with and then lead to the fulfillment of your vision.

## Chapter Twelve

# Finding the Right Members for Your Team

**Nothing is more critical to the ultimate success of a dental office than the selection of the individuals who comprise the dental team.** The creation of an inspiring vision, and even the most vivid sharing of same, will do no good if the people that form your team are, by their very nature, not receptive to the particular values and goals this vision entails. It is possible to make some minor changes in the behavior of team members through training and from the effects of your office vision. It is not possible to change the basic character of the individuals you employ, so hiring the correct people is imperative.

The information that follows is desperately needed by our lonely solo pilot, but everyone in our profession will at some point need to add or replace staff. Knowing how to effectively select the people you'll be entering the daily dental wars with is vital to your **success** and **happiness!** Nothing is more distressing than being forced to work each day with people whose values you don't share and whom you don't enjoy—be you doctor or auxiliary.

The keys to finding the right people to fulfill your office vision are:

1. Precisely identify the attributes in others that your professional vision mandates for the development of the office of your dreams.
2. Create a hiring process that, when followed, will make the virtues you esteem obvious in the people you are evaluating.
3. Consistently observe that process in staff selection.

Remember, no amount of effort or patience in staff training, nor the most sophisticated of staff meetings, can replace the essential task of hiring the right person in the first place.

Let's examine a hypothetical situation (which, of course, really happened to me), and see if we can illustrate these points more clearly. Suppose you purchase an office with two chairsides who have been employed there for a number of years. One is both punctual and reliable. She works hard at her job and is dexterous and efficient.

But a significant part of the values you have identified for your dream office deals with relating to the patient as a whole person, not just a mouth containing teeth to be "worked on." To attain these objectives will require the development of a high-trust relationship that allows for an open and forthright dialogue between your staff and patients. This type of meaningful conversation will enable both you and your team to help patients clarify their personal values as regards their own dental health. Thus, through this personal relationship, your office is better able to help the patients you care for to both select and achieve the level of dental health appropriate for them at this point in time.

In this new awareness, you notice that your assistant—that pinnacle of chairside efficiency—is rather cold and abrupt with patients. She seems annoyed by questions, and likes to hurry clients out of the operatory, to accelerate the preparation of the treatment area for the next procedure.

The second chairside you inherited is not outstandingly efficient. She likes to visit with patients, and doesn't work as quickly as her fellow assistant. This pattern of behavior annoyed you on your busy first days, but now you notice how the patients frequently ask her questions. For some reason they ask her about their dental condition, even after you have left the treatment area—your scholarly explanation of their needed care still hanging freshly in the vapors. In light of your newly identified values, you see this knack of answering patient questions is essential for the creation of the high-trust relationships you are trying to establish with your clients.

In this scenario we have identified a difference in values between the two staff people we've discussed. Depending on the criteria of excellence established by the team leader, ONE of these assistants will be judged as outstanding, and the other as wanting. But which individual is perceived to be outstanding is totally the opinion of the person doing the judging. What you must see is that neither person's actions are right or wrong—good or bad. They are simply behaving in a way consistent with their own personal beliefs.

The first assistant we described values hard work and efficiency. She's not too comfortable with people, but prefers to concentrate her efforts on the skillful performance of tasks. Her strengths include the ability to produce prodigious amounts of work, and her reliability.

Our second staff member is a people person. She has good skills chairside, but she comes to work to be with people and help them, not simply to pass instruments. It is the conversation and company she values and enjoys. The work of assisting is something she tolerates while receiving her enjoyment from the people who surround her.

I don't believe it is possible to transmute the character of one assistant into the other, no matter how hard you try. I believe that an effort to change the nature of people leads only to frustration on the part of everyone involved. You have three choices in this situation.

1. You can continue as you are, and face the growing tension that comes from conflicts in values and poor communications.

2. You can reassign the assistant whose values don't coincide with yours to a job that will accent her strengths and hide what you now perceive to be her weakness. Possibly a front office or clerical position, that requires great concentration and accuracy with less patient interaction, would make our hard-working but not people-oriented chairside once again a valued staff member. For your "people person," perhaps the ideal position would be in case presentation, or the delicate job of collections, that requires tact more than efficiency and could be more suited to her natural temperament.
3. The third choice is to tell your staff member she is not the right person for the job she currently holds (she'll know already), and support her as she searches for another position where she very well may become that office's "star."

I hope this illustration has made clear the essential need to have worked through your own office vision before any steps of the hiring process have begun. Let's return now to the plight of our solo dentist. While the decision to retain, retrain or dismiss an existing staff member is vital to the happiness and success of every office—our poor hero has no staff! Allow me to carefully guide you through my own system of identifying new team members.

The process we use in our office for hiring staff is deliberate and demanding. It requires a lot of time and effort. In our office we have one staff member who has been with us since a few months after the office opened, 20 years ago. The average length of employment of our current staff is about six years. This average is decreased by the fact that we have grown and added additional staff.

My point is, the process of hiring the right people repays you many times over, because you won't have to begin the search for new staff again every three months, when you realize the last person you selected isn't going to work out. Also, there exists but little conflict, and a great deal of joy, in working every day with people who share your beliefs and values.

Let us go carefully through all the steps that our hiring procedure entails. I assure you that every time we add staff, this is the exact process we follow—point by painstaking point. Let the complexity and detail of this process testify to how important the selection of the right staff is to the success of our office.

Before we enter the hiring arena, allow me to beg your indulgence on one point. In all the years I have been in practice I have had one male applicant for a staff position (he wasn't qualified). In this lengthy chapter I will refer to all applicants as female in gender. I do this only to simplify the writing process. In my two years in the military I am proud to say I served with many excellent male auxiliaries. I hope to see an increase in male ancillary staffing. We need all the good people we can get in our profession. Unfortunately, in Keokuk, I know of no males employed in any area offices.

The first and most critical step in our hiring process is to attract a large pool of outstanding applicants. We need our recruiting process to reach out to people who share our values, no matter in what field of employment they have previously worked. We would like our efforts to yield applications from individuals who previously believed they would never consider working for a dentist.

In our rural area, I seldom have more than two or three people apply for an available staff position with previous dental experience or training. To allow us the greatest possible chance of finding the ideal person to join our team, we MUST recruit applicants from outside the normal group of individuals that might consider a dental office as a possible place of employment. For example, in the past, two people with teaching degrees have graced our office with their presence.

Our process of initially attracting new staff revolves principally around help-wanted ads, placed in every local paper within a 20-mile radius of our office. We have no dental assistant association, or assistant school near us to approach as a possible source of job applicants. If we were fortunate enough to have either resource available to us, they would be the first entities I would contact in my search for additional team members.

Anything you can do to increase the numbers of potential staff members that apply for work with your team is to the good. There may well be opportunities for you to explore in your location that don't exist in ours.

Our staff has a standing offer of a $100 bonus for identifying a potential staff person that we hire. I personally keep my eyes open for patients, waitresses, bank tellers, or anyone else I feel may possess the qualities we esteem.

In our rural area, 90-plus percent of the applicant pool our office attracts comes from the help-wanted ad that follows. Thus the make-up and character of the ad your office will place is critical. This notice must accurately identify the VALUES you seek in your future staff member, as you wish your message to appeal to people who share similar beliefs to those you and your team hold. For our office, the following advertisement performs this task. Your office ad must vary to reflect your own unique values.

---

DENTAL TEAM: Are you kind, compassionate, people-oriented, and motivated to succeed? We are seeking an exceptional person for our progressive office. We value superior organizational and administrative skills and we focus on warmth, caring, and expert communication with our clients. We emphasize personal development through continuing education, full participation with the other members of our team and high involvement with our clients. Although previous experience in dentistry is not essential, we believe that applicants should be career-minded, personally stable, and health-centered in their lifestyle. If you are searching for a real opportunity to grow and fulfill your potential, please send a complete resume to:

Dr. John A. Wilde, D.D.S., P.C.
1610 Morgan Street
Keokuk, Iowa 52632.

*(We end this copy with instructions to every newspaper within a 20-mile radius of our office to:)* Please place this in your paper for one week.

Thank you.
John A. Wilde D.D.S., P.C.

---

Sure, our ad is lengthy and expensive to run. It costs a lot more than "Wanted—Dental Assistant." The effort to create this ad and the expense to run it merely buttress my statement of belief in the critical need to find and employ the best possible team members.

I'd like to point out two salient features of our ad. The first is that the entire description of the person we are searching for is based on values. The second is that we have none of the NORMAL stuff usually listed about potential jobs in our advertisement. Nothing that says good hours, salary, or benefits. Our position provides all those things, but to state these facets of our available job won't appeal to the values held by the people we are trying to identify.

We are not seeking to hire people whose main motivation to work is to obtain the "things" they are given for their job performance.

We seek people who are kind and compassionate to others. We want applicants who are already exceptional and want to grow. It's wonderful if they have worked in a dental office previously, but we're more concerned about their innate character. Do they share the values that we believe in and try to share with our clients? Would I hire a smoker? Unlikely. That behavior illustrates to me values not consistent with those held by our staff.

We make compromises, of course. This ad is our best effort to identify the personal beliefs my team admires. We don't all live up to these values every moment of our lives, but they represent our goals. Do you see why value clarification is so essential before you can begin the hiring process? *Values for us are the hiring process.* In other words, in our office hiring consists of identifying the values we want in a new staff member, and finding someone who shares those values. Once we find the right person, we'll be able to teach them to perform the tasks required of them.

This ad also keeps some folks away. The people whose only question about an available position is, "How much does it pay?" aren't attracted by this notice. We rarely have a smoker even apply. The two things we wish ideally to achieve through this publication are to:

1. Maximize the flow of applications from like-valued people.
2. Minimize the applications from folks, no matter how delightful, who don't qualify as team members of our office and thus save everyone some wasted time.

Don't copy this ad. Create a unique statement that helps you to proceed in your own value clarification process. Ask "What do we desire from this new staff member?" Not just what tasks must they perform, but what kind of a person do we seek? The answer to these questions defines your ad.

Your ad has been placed and the resumes come rolling in. Depending on the local economy and time of year, we will receive between 30 and 70 applications, each of which I review personally.

Some I eliminate out of hand. I get rid of the ones written in pencil or from recent high school graduates, unless something in their resume leads me to believe they have a clearly thought-out set of values. I am lenient at this stage of our process, however. Anyone I eliminate now will be dropped from all further consideration. If there is *any chance*, in my estimation, of the candidate having potential, I pass this person on to the next portion of our hiring procedure.

This next step consists of a patterned telephone interview. Within our office, this step is always performed by a senior staff member, usually the most senior in the department (hygiene, chairside or front office) to which we will be adding the new employee. Beginning dentists must, of course, complete each step themselves, unless they have a spouse with the interest and ability to assist them.

I say patterned interview as the same employee asks identical questions to each applicant. This is a time-consuming task and we have to free the staff person doing the telephone interviews from the tasks that would normally occupy their day for a considerable amount of time. We must allow them whatever freedom may be required to carefully accomplish this important segment of our hiring process. Take a moment and review the form used for this step of our selection process.

---

## Telephone Interview

Name: ____________________

Address: ____________________

Phone: Home____________ Office ____________

How long have you lived at your current address? ____________

How often have you moved in the last 5 years? ____________

Do you have reliable transportation available?_____What? ________

What hours are you available to work?

Full-time Part-time Evenings Saturday

What salary do you expect? ____________

When would you be available to start working? ____________

Are you currently employed?______Where?____________

Can we contact them?______What is your job title? ____________

How long have you worked there?____________

Previous job held__________Reason for leaving ____________

Have you been absent many days during the past years? ________

Why? ____________________

Do you smoke?_______

Is there a reason why you couldn't pass a physical exam? ________

Is there someone you consider your dentist? ____________

What condition do you consider your teeth and gums to be in? ______

How often do you visit a dentist? ____________

What was the highest grade you completed in school?____________

Have you had any college or advanced training? ____________

What hobbies or interests do you have? ____________

Are you a member of any civic, professional or social organization?

____________________

What are your plans for the next 5 years? ____________

TELEPHONE IMPRESSIONS: Excellent Good Fair Poor

Capacity to communicate: ____________________

Voice: ____________________

Clarity of expression: ____________________

Ease of expression: ____________________

---

The person conducting the interview needs to take a few minutes to explain the purpose of this call, which is to get to know the applicant, gather some information and answer any questions she may have. The tone set with the applicant should be friendly and relaxed—even fun. The questions start with requests for some simple facts that we probably already have available from the resume the applicant has sent us. We need to allow a little time for the candidates to relax and be at their best. Answering these early factual questions provides this opportunity.

I think the reason for us acquiring most of the factual information is self-evident. You will see as we proceed that we concentrate a great deal of our attention on the personal dental awareness of the applicant. In my past experience, hiring someone with no history of valuing good oral health has proven to be a big mistake. No matter how strong the applicant's other features may be, if they have been to the dentist only once in the last five years, and that for treatment of a toothache, they have almost no chance of being invited for a personal interview.

Some of you may feel that this deficiency in dental values by the applicant can be overcome by proper education, if the candidate has other excellent qualities. This may be true, but it has decidedly NOT been the case in my experience. I believe the questions concerning the applicant's dental history are really inquiries into this individual's personal values and feelings concerning the level of commitment to personal well-being.

Hobbies are important if you wish to hire a chairside. Most people with good hand-eye coordination find ways to use this skill. It may be knitting, sewing, or playing the piano, but there is usually some indication of this innate coordination in the applicant's choice of hobbies. (Personally, I like to read. If you saw an amalgam I had carved, I think you would agree this supports my thesis that eye-hand coordination will be revealed by a choice of activities selected. At least I do turn my own pages.)

I prefer to employ people that are involved socially. They represent the "people-oriented" kind of staff we are searching for. Leadership in organizations is even more impressive, as it shows they are committed to their activities, and are acknowledged as leaders by their peers.

As for their imminent plans, if they share with us that they wish to have a baby or return to school in the near future, this job isn't for them. The best assistant in the world does me no good if she is no longer employed in my office.

All this information is helpful, but we gather a lot of the same data on the application form we'll discuss next. The MOST CRITICAL function of this interview is the *personal impression made by the applicant on the individual conducting the interview.* If the applicants come off badly in the appraisal, they have little chance of proceeding in the hiring process. If they sound flat, dull and lifeless on the phone now, I certainly don't want them to represent our office.

The most essential section of the telephone interview which is of critical import in the selection process, is the TELEPHONE IMPRESSION SECTION AT THE VERY END OF THE FORM. It is here that I ask my staff for that critical intangible: their judgment. The impression made by the applicant on my skilled staff member—or on our solo doctor or his or her spouse—during this lengthy conversation is much more important to me than any factual data we may have recorded.

If the candidate passes this stage of the hiring process they are invited to our office, and asked to fill out the personal record form seen below. This is completed by the applicant in our reception room during office hours. If at all possible, the filling out of this form is scheduled at a time when the same staff person who did the phone interview is present. Thus the applicant is greeted by an "old friend."

When the candidates present themselves to complete the personal record form, they are again evaluated by the staff. I believe this evaluation to be more meaningful if done by the same individual who has engaged in the phone conversation with them recently. When they arrived to fill out the application, were they pleasant and friendly? Did they have a nice smile? Was their appearance neat and professional? We don't desire to hire beauty queens, but we do want staff members who represent our values of good health, and show a positive self-image by looking neat and professional. How attractive God happened to make them doesn't matter to us at all. We are concerned with the VALUES they display in their behavior and demeanor.

I can't over-stress the importance I place on staff evaluation of candidates. The formal interview process that I will conduct is stressful and takes place in an artificial environment. So often the true qualities of a person, good or bad, are more accurately revealed in these less formal relations with my staff. Applicants will let their hair down and ask questions of the staff they would never dream of asking in the interview. This knowledge, gained through the perception of experienced team members, is priceless in the selection process.

The staff member's impressions are recorded on a corner of the application form in red pen. These notes usually consist of a few words, such as "pleasant, nice smile, asked good questions." Or possibly, "Didn't seem friendly, very casually dressed, smile not attractive."

---

## Personal Record Form

Please be as complete as possible. All information you give here will be held in *strict confidence.*

Name__________________________________ Date ______________

Address __________________________________________________

Previous Address ___________________________________________

Home Phone______________ Social Security Number ______________

Earnings Expected __________________________________________

WORK EXPERIENCE: Please start with your present or most recent position.

I. Employer ______________ Address ________________________

Business phone ____________ Employed from ________ to ________

Kind of work ____________ Your title ________________________

Nature of your work ________________________________________

Skills acquired ____________________________________________

Salary or salary range ______________________________________

Supervisory responsibility ________ Immed. Superior ____________

What do you enjoy best about your job? ______________________

____________________________________________________________

What do you enjoy least about your job? ______________________

____________________________________________________________

Reason for leaving (or desiring a change)? ____________________

____________________________________________________________

II. Employer ________________________________________________

Address ____________________________________________________

Business phone ____________ Employed from ________ to ________

Kind of work ____________ Your title ________________________

Nature of your work ________________________________________

Skills acquired ____________________________________________

Salary or salary range ______________________________________

Supervisory responsibility ________ Immed. Superior ____________

What do you enjoy best about your job? ______________________

____________________________________________________________

What do you enjoy least about your job? ______________________

____________________________________________________________

Reason for leaving (or desiring a change)? ____________________

____________________________________________________________

III. Employer _______________________________________________

Address ____________________________________________________

Business phone ____________ Employed from ________ to ________

Kind of work ____________ Your title ________________________

Nature of your work ________________________________________

Skills acquired ____________________________________________

Salary or salary range ______________________________________

Supervisory responsibility ________ Immed. Superior ____________

What do you enjoy best about your job? ________________________

________________________________________________

What do you enjoy least about your job? ________________________

________________________________________________

Reason for leaving? ________________________________

________________________________________________

Other positions held? ______________________________

Indicate by number any of the above employers you do not wish contacted. ________________________________

## ACTIVITIES AND INTERESTS

Membership in civic, professional or social organizations __________

________________________________________________

What hobbies interest you? __________________________

Why did you apply for this position? ____________________

________________________________________________

In what way do you feel qualified for this position? ____________

________________________________________________

What are your plans for the future? ______________________

________________________________________________

Why do you work? ________________________________

What starting salary would you expect? ____________________

What income would you desire to enable you to live as you would like to live? ________________________________

PLEASE LIST THREE REFERENCES:

| | Names | Addresses | Phone Numbers |
|---|---|---|---|
| 1 | ____________ | ____________ | ____________ |
| | ____________ | ____________ | ____________ |
| 2 | ____________ | ____________ | ____________ |
| | ____________ | ____________ | ____________ |
| 3 | ____________ | ____________ | ____________ |
| | ____________ | ____________ | ____________ |

## PHYSICAL DATA

List any serious illness, operation, accident, or nervous disorder you have had with approximate dates ________________________

What allergies do you have? ______________________________

What medications do you take? ____________________________

What brand of cigarettes do you smoke?________Why?____________

Would a job that required you to be on your feet all day be objectionable?

______________________________________________________

Would assisting at a surgical operation bother you? _____________

Would you be willing to have a complete medical and dental exam, with a report filed to this office?______________________________

What three characteristics best describe you? __________________

______________________________________________________

What short and long term goals do you personally have? __________

______________________________________________________

______________________________________________________

______________________________________________________

______________________________________________________

**EDUCATION**

Indicate highest grade completed:

| | | | | | | | | |
|---|---|---|---|---|---|---|---|---|
| Elementary | 6 | 7 | 8 | | | | | |
| High School | 1 | 2 | 3 | 4 | | | | |
| College | 1 | 2 | 3 | 4 | 5 | 6 | 7 | 8 |

Approximate grade point average ___________________________

Approximate number in high school class _____________________

Approximate class standing________________________________

Favorite high school subjects ______________________________

Least liked_____________________________________________

Extra-curricular activities _________________________________

______________________________________________________

Part-time and summer work ________________________________

Class and other offices held ________________________________

Colleges attended and dates attended _______________________

______________________________________________________

Major fields_____________________________________________

Degree(s) and year(s) obtained ______________________________

Extra-curricular activities _________________________________

______________________________________________________

How was your education financed? ______________________________

% expenses you earned? ______________________________________

Part-time and summer work in college? __________________________

_____________________________________________________________

**MY DENTAL HISTORY**

Is there someone that you consider as "your" dentist:? ____________

If you were asked to refer someone to a dentist, do you know of one whom you would choose?__________Why? ____________________

If you have changed dentists in the last five years, please indicate:

Yes_____ No_____

Circumstances and reasons ____________________________________

Do you consider your teeth and oral structure to be in:

Excellent_____ Good_____ Fair_____ Poor_____ condition?

Were your dental services during the past five years thorough and very complete? Yes_____ No_____

How often have you visited a dentist in the past five years? _________

How often did you visit the dentist for preventive examinations?

Every 3 months_____ Every year_____

Every 6 months_____ Other_____

If other, please indicate ______________________________________

What services were performed on these visits? ___________________

_____________________________________________________________

Was there any treatment that was suggested but not performed? ______

_____________________________________________________________

Was this due to any specific reason? ____________________________

My opinion about dentistry is different from other people's because: __

_____________________________________________________________

This is an exact copy of the application form we use in our office. I believe (also hope and pray) we are violating none of the laws covering fairness and equity in the hiring process. Please feel free to adopt or modify our form for your own use, as you see fit. You **must** ask your attorney, or someone from your state job service, to review the form before using it, to assure that you haven't inadvertently broken one of the myriad and constantly changing regulations concerning what can and cannot be asked of a potential employee.

I have a strong urge to editorialize, possibly to pontificate, on government interference in the hiring process. I guess there is no point to such comments, as the regulations that currently exist won't be changed due to any thoughts of mine. Do be advised that violating these fair employment laws can result in severe penalties. Be certain that whatever form you use is in complete compliance with all state and federal mandates concerning hiring.

The first line of our Personal Record Form states that all the information submitted to us in trust will be held in *strict confidence*. To those of you with existing staff, be sure that everyone involved in the hiring process respects and understands this commitment. The confidentiality that is promised is your ethical responsibility to insure. As with patient confidentiality, this is not a matter to be taken lightly. Be sure that your team is clear that no discussion of the information gathered in the hiring process can ever be allowed outside the office.

The first paragraph of the form asks the applicants to give you an estimate of the level of compensation they would expect, if this position is attained. The information gained from this query is somewhat difficult to interpret.

If a potential team member lists minimum wage for expected earnings, it could indicate a low self-esteem. It could also mean that they really desire the job as described in the advertisement, and money is not a primary motivating factor for them. If they request a figure doubling the salary you are able to offer, it is possible you won't be able to afford to hire them. However, over the years I've offered a position to people at a much lower salary than they had quoted as "earnings expected" and had them accept the job. This figure may give you some insight into the person applying, but use this single bit of data carefully and in combination with other information you acquire.

I wouldn't eliminate a candidate solely on the basis of this response, no matter what desired earnings they state. If the salary figure quoted is well above what the position available would pay, but you are impressed with the applicant, I would suggest when you, your spouse or staff member calls to schedule an interview, inform the applicant of the range of possible salaries. If this is acceptable to them, schedule the interview. If it isn't, thank the applicant for their interest and move on in the hiring process. You've saved everyone a lot of time and trouble.

In reviewing the "history of work experience" section of our personal record form, I look carefully for a pattern of ***too much job mobility.*** No matter what reasons for switching jobs are given, a person who historically has moved from employer to employer probably won't be in your office long either. I think you'll often find the reason given for past career movement has something to do with "unfair treatment" in previous jobs. This, at least, is the applicant's perception and/or explanation.

My guess is, should you employ them, they will feel unfairly treated by you before long. The two exceptions to my negative perception of job mobility are career advancement opportunities, or a geographic move that requires a change in employment. I am even suspicious of these incidents. Good people tend to find the right employment situation and remain in it.

In addition to stability in past employment, I look for patterns of upward mobility within previous jobs—both in salary and responsibility. Evidence of advances in either is very impressive to me.

As is the case with my review of the entire form, I analyze this section for *completeness* of answers and *quality of expression.* Many job applicants don't even bother to fully complete all of our admittedly (and deliberately) long form. If they lack the commitment to thoroughly fill out an application, how well do you believe they will perform if they secure the job? I also like to study the applicant's use of language in answering our questions. I believe a form that could be answered with yes or no responses would greatly reduce my ability to see into the mind of an applicant.

Be certain, when you arrive at the point in your hiring process that involves reference checks, that you are cognizant of any employers the applicant has asked you on the application NOT to contact. If it was a *previous employer* the applicant doesn't want notified, I'd like to know why we shouldn't communicate with them and would listen very carefully to the candidate's explanation. Is there a chance that something occurred on that job that our potential team member doesn't want us to be aware of?

However, never risk a applicant's current job by contacting the employer without permission. Sometimes the employer is aware of their plans to leave the business and will prove an excellent source of information. Be very certain this is the case before speaking with them. I would hate to be responsible, legally or morally, for the dismissal of a job applicant due to an unauthorized inquiry from my staff.

Under the Activities and Interests section of the form, we again ask what starting salary they would expect if selected for the position. Very often the figure listed here varies from the one recorded on the first page of the application or given during our telephone interview. You may wish to question this inconsistency.

You will see a good number of questions duplicated in the different parts of our hiring process. This is not carelessness or an error on our part. I am always amazed at the different answers given to the same question, asked at different times and places in our employment routine. Sometimes this variation may simply indicate the applicant has had time to consider the matter more carefully. Other times it will reveal a tendency to be "creative" with the truth.

As we mentioned earlier during our discussion of the phone interview, hobbies and activities that our applicant participates in can provide us with some very useful information. Questions such as "What are you plans for the future?" and "Why do you work?" help us to identify values and goals of the applicants, as well as displaying their ability to express themselves.

Under Physical Data, I wish to identify smokers, and be sure all candidates are physically able to perform the job. Many years ago—before we had developed our current application form—I hired a chairside who couldn't stand to watch us give local anesthetic. She had a three-day career in our office. (By the end of the three fateful days she had backed so far away from the treatment areas that she was out in the street!) Better for both of us if we had identified her distress at any "surgical procedure" before employing her.

We ask every applicant if they are "willing to have a complete medical and dental exam?" We won't require it, but if they answer NO, I want an explanation. A friend of mine once hired a chairside with early MS. It was a sad situation for everyone involved when they all realized she wasn't capable of handling the tasks required of her.

The questions on personal goals and a self-description of the applicants again give you a chance to examine their values and writing ability. As you can see, I like to scatter the questions that provide me with information about the person, and not just their factual history, throughout the form. I believe this provides more insight than lumping all similar questions in one area.

Under the education section of the application, I want to see what level of training and/or formal education they have achieved, of course. I enjoy the company of intelligent and well-educated people, and this information helps me to identify them. (Note, I didn't say I was one, I just said that I enjoy their company.) I'm also interested in their work ethic. A detailed account of summer jobs and methods used in helping to pay for college expenses often illustrates the type of ambition and fortitude I admire in a fellow employee.

We have touched on my feeling about the critical importance of the dental history as an indicator for potential success as an employee in my office. Please forgive my redundancy, but I would give this section of the application your most careful evaluation. I have had applicants that were excellent in every area we considered except their dental values. I have hired them in spite of this shortcoming and have been sorry every time. I think a lot of you will minimize the importance of this factor as a predictor of employment success (as I once did). If you do, I'm pretty sure you'll come to regret it.

At this point, we have all the factual data we will gather. I now review the information we have obtained during the entire process and select the people I will be personally interviewing.

I lean heavily on my staff evaluations, both concerning the phone interview and their observations of potential team members as applications were being filled out in our office reception area. I have in the past ignored their input and scheduled an interview with an applicant who "looks good on paper," but whom my staff had rated poorly. Usually I know the person isn't right for the job two minutes after we begin our discussion. In this unfortunate scenario, we have wasted not only my time, and the applicant's, but the effort and talent of the team member whose judgment I have ignored.

After a thorough review of all the data we have collected, I usually select from six to eight people to interview. I set aside one hour to spend with each candidate. We try to schedule everyone within the time frame of a few days if possible. I tend to forget some details of our discussion, no matter how carefully I take notes, if too long a time passes between the initial and final interview of all our candidates. The impressions made by the most recently spoken to applicants are so much stronger than those made by candidates interviewed a week earlier that the entire interview process can be biased.

The choice to do all the interviews as closely together as possible often means an entire day will be devoted to the task. Staff are so critical to the success of any practice that a day devoted to nothing but interviews is a small price to pay considering the value to be gained.

I have been forced, by the limited availability of a candidate, to conduct interviews in the evening, after work. I think this is unfair both to the interviewer and to the applicant, as neither of you are at your best. I interview at the end of a working day only if no other physical possibility for us to meet within my established time frame exists.

The personal interview is a critical step in the hiring process. Everything possible must be done to maximize its effectiveness. Please remember, dentists aren't trained to interview prospective employees, and most of us are probably only fair (at best) in this subtle art. Knowing this, we must do everything possible to assure ourselves of the best chance to gain the most valuable and least biased information from the interview.

Before I greet each applicant, I will have again reviewed ALL the forms that have been filled out to date, and completed what parts of the SUMMARY FORM (contained later in this chapter) I could, based on the information we have gathered prior to the interview. I will make a written list of any unique concerns or question I want to ask a particular candidate. When I am confident my preparation for this interview is complete, I will go to our reception room and personally greet the individual waiting for me.

I always shake hands and introduce myself to the interviewee. The degree of "cold and clammy" I find in the grip tells me the level of apprehension that exists. This tension is my enemy, as it can hide the best qualities of some excellent individuals. I don't wish to hire someone who is skilled at the art of interviewing, but to evaluate them as a potential team member. I want each applicant relaxed and at their best during this interview process.

It is a major responsibility of the interviewer to allow whatever time is needed to create an environment where the applicant can relax and accurately display her finest attributes. This isn't dissimilar to the beginning of all new patient interviews, also done in my private office. A relaxed, pleasant, informal atmosphere is most conducive to the outcome we desire in both new patient and job applicant interview situations.

I invite the candidate to be seated in my office. We will not be disturbed for any reason (short of fire in the building!) during this interview. I begin by thanking them for making the effort to apply, and for their interest in our office. I truly am grateful. Often I compliment them on their appearance, and we chat a few minutes on whatever neutral topic seems appropriate, from weather to mutual friends and interests. I already know a lot about them from reviewing our already completed forms, so finding a topic to begin our discussion is simple.

My staff has checked our computer, and if the applicant has been seen in our office as a patient, I have their dental records available. It's unfortunate (and embarrassing!) to begin an interview by introducing yourself to an existing patient as if they were a stranger.

Once I sense by their tone and body language that they have relaxed, I begin the formal interview. I start by apologizing. I explain that I don't interview often, and due to my deficiencies as an interviewer, I will ask them the same series of "patterned" questions that I ask each applicant. I add that I feel asking each person the identical questions gives a more equitable outcome to the interview process. I also mention that I will take some notes during their responses, and please don't be distracted by my scribbling.

I assure the interviewee the queries I will ask have no right or wrong answer, but are simply intended to help me get to know them. I encourage them to ask me questions at any time. We then proceed to the patterned interview.

I tend to talk too much. This is ALWAYS a mistake, but it is a deadly sin in an interview. (My M.D. brother Jim recently informed me that:

1. You never lose weight eating, and
2. You never learn anything while talking. Both bits of advice seem accurate, but I have no idea why he happened to share this wealth of the obvious with me!)

The patterned question format helps limit my tendency to wax, if not eloquent, at least verbose. I used to spend a lot of time explaining the job details during the interview. That got tedious, even for a self-confessed "talker." The following Job Benefit Description I hand to the interviewee when they first ask a question about working conditions. I give them a minute to peruse this document, and answer any concerns they may have. Not only does the job description form save time, but in case there exists a misunderstanding concerning benefits at a later date, we have this standard document we reviewed together available as a reference.

When we complete the hiring process, we require each new staff member to review our office policy manual, and sign a statement that she has read and understands its content. The objective is again to eliminate any potential misunderstandings about the specific benefits and requirements of employment on our office team. This manual contains in much greater detail all the information concerning employment conditions and regulations in our office. The brief job description used only during interviews is simply a "shorthand" version, to save our precious interview time.

## Job Benefit Description

- THREE-MONTH PROBATIONARY PERIOD BEFORE BENEFITS BECOME EFFECTIVE.
- STARTING SALARY $6 to $9 AN HOUR DEPENDING ON THE LEVEL OF PREVIOUS EXPERIENCE.
- SIX PAID HOLIDAYS A YEAR.
- ONE WEEK PAID VACATION AFTER ONE YEAR OF EMPLOYMENT.
- TWO WEEKS PAID VACATION AFTER TWO YEARS OF EMPLOYMENT.
- HEALTH BONUS—1/2 DAY PAID SICK LEAVE PER MONTH. IF EMPLOYEES DO NOT USE THEIR SICK DAYS, THEY RECEIVE THIS BENEFIT IN SALARY.
- ALL UNIFORMS PURCHASED BY OFFICE.
- WORKMEN'S COMPENSATION INSURANCE.
- CONTINUING EDUCATION—ALL EXPENSES AND SALARY PAID ON NORMAL WORKING DAYS.
- ALL DENTAL WORK FREE TO STAFF EXCEPT FOR LAB BILLS. TWENTY-FIVE PERCENT OFF ALL DENTAL CARE FOR OTHER FAMILY MEMBERS.

## Patterned Personal Interview

1. What are three things you do to promote your good health? ______
   ______
2. What do you do to promote your own dental health? ______
   ______
3. What quality do you value most in other people? ______
   ______
4. What kind of persons do you prefer to work with? ______
   ______
5. What is most important to you in a job? ______
   What do you care least about in a job? ______
6. What job do you wish to have in five years? ______
7. How do you react when you are asked to work overtime? ______
   ______
8. What additional training do you feel you need to realize your career goals? ______
9. Would you rather be assigned a task and be responsible for it or do you prefer to work with someone else at all times? ______
   Why? ______
10. What situations have you found most stressful on the job? ______
    ______
    What techniques have you found to manage these stresses? ______
    ______
11. What words do other people use to describe you? ______
12. If you have a variety of tasks which you need to accomplish in a given period of time, what approach do you take? ______
13. How do you react when treated unfairly in an everyday situation?
    ______
14. How do you feel about taking on additional responsibility? ______
    ______
15. What impression do you think you create with other people? ______
    ______
16. What plans do you have for your own personal improvement? ______
    ______
17. Of what three accomplishments are you most proud? ______
    ______

18. How have your past job experiences prepared you for this position?
________________________________________
19. What is your interpretation of "success"? ____________________
20. If you could structure the perfect job for yourself, what would you do and why?____________________________________

I don't believe I've ever asked all the questions on this patterned interview to any one applicant. The form functions as a guide to lead the conversation. The purpose isn't to fill out this paper, but to determine if the individual I'm currently interviewing will be an asset to our team. I have some specific questions prepared especially for this individual, based on the application information we have previously gathered. Usually I will make these queries after the patterned interview is completed, when the maximum understanding between us has been established.

I believe by now, you possess enough information on our hiring system to evaluate the style and purpose of the patterned interview questions. They are again all open-ended questions, to encourage the applicant to speak. The aim of each question is to identify values more than to establish facts. As this discussion proceeds I evaluate the applicant for an overall impression too. Is she poised? How is her grammar? Do you notice a sense of humor present? *Is this someone you would enjoy working with?*

The patterned questions begin by requesting relatively easy, factual information, and then grow more abstract. You will wish to develop your own interview questions based on the values you and your team have identified. That is as it should be. My emphasis here is not to discuss the particular questions of our form, but to provide an example and establish the benefits of a patterned interview format.

We end the interview promptly at the scheduled time. I ask if there are any questions our applicant has that I may answer. When these are responded to, I thank our candidate again for her time, and promise to notify her as soon as we have reached a hiring decision. I think immediate notification of the outcome of the hiring process is the least you owe these people for the time they have invested with you. This promise of notification also saves us time by preventing each candidate from calling the office and "quizzing" the staff about how close we are to reaching a final decision.

Over the years a number of new patient families have come from people we interviewed and didn't hire. Please remember that the hiring process represents your office as certainly as every other function your team performs. These applicants are judging you and your staff, even as you evaluate them, and their opinion will be carried to the community. As always, we wish the impression our office leaves with people to be a positive one.

As soon as my office door has closed behind the applicant, I begin to fill out our Summary Form. I allow myself 10 minutes of the allotted hour interview period for this task and to review the information for the next scheduled interview. Much of the summary form is already completed from information gathered before meeting the applicant, but I want to record pertinent facts about our discussion while it is completely fresh in my mind, and not after six more interviews have taken place. The information condensed on our summary form will be critical in helping me reach a final hiring decision.

---

## Summary Form

Name: ____________________________________________

Age: __________ (Author's note: This is my estimation of their age only. I can look and guess, but not legally or in good taste ask.)

Application letter: ____________________________________

____________________________________________

____________________________________________

Appearance and voice: __________________________________

____________________________________________

Work history (skills and experience): ______________________

____________________________________________

____________________________________________

Motivation to work; aims in life; achievement of goals: ___________

______________________________________________

______________________________________________

Health: chronic disease, days missed last year: ____________

______________________________________________

Education: ______________________________________

Dental history: __________________________________

______________________________________________

Family background: marriage, parents and siblings, children: ______

______________________________________________

Family support for working: _______________________

Social background: ______________________________

Activities enjoyed: ______________________________

Leadership: ____________________________________

Test scores: ___________________________________

Reference check: _______________________________

______________________________________________

______________________________________________

Comments: job strengths and weaknesses: ______________

______________________________________________

______________________________________________

Recommendations: ______________________________

______________________________________________

______________________________________________

When the interviewing is completed, I sit down with a hot cup of coffee, and once again truncate our list of possible candidates. Usually by this point in the process we will have from two to four candidates remaining under consideration. Sometimes I have one candidate that seems clearly superior to all other applicants. If that is so, I will proceed to our final hiring steps with her alone involved. If in these final steps a question of her suitability arises, I will go back and review the information on our other finalists.

More frequently there will be two or three fairly equal applicants. If that is the case all of them will remain involved in the final segments of our hiring process.

The next step in our selection process is to check references on each remaining candidate. The reference checks are CRITICAL. They are also difficult and tricky to do. They are performed by the same senior staff member who did the phone interviews. Often our best information comes from fellow workers at a previous job. Our technique is to call the previous places of employment we have received permission to contact and ask to speak to someone who worked with our candidate.

We seldom contact the references listed by the candidate, on the theory that anyone can find three people who like you. We use these sources only if we aren't allowed access to previous places of employment. We try to get *three* completed reference checks on each applicant still under consideration.

NEVER FAIL TO CHECK REFERENCES. It can save you from embezzlement and many other potential headaches, as well as greatly augment the information you possess on each applicant. Frequently a very strong, or a very weak reference, will sway the final hiring decision.

An area dentist was sued for sexual harassment by an employee a few years ago. The charges made the front page of our local paper. Later the doctor found this lady had a history of such allegations at two previous jobs. Do you think he regretted not doing a more thorough reference check?

If a reference check is requested of us by a potential employer of a past member of our team, we reveal only the dates of employment of the former staff person, and their beginning and ending compensation. That is it! To do more puts you at risk of potential litigation. All of my staff are carefully instructed in this regard, as even if the call they get concerning references on a former employee is received at their home, I am legally responsible for their responses.

Please call the employment department of any industry around you and ask for information about former employees. Dates of employment and beginning and final salary are all the information you will be given. If you decide to help a dentist buddy and provide more information (which I have done), at least be aware that you are opening yourself to potential legal action.

Good news! Most dentists are too uninformed to know this, and will just blabber away about a previous employee. One told me he wouldn't touch the B—— with a 10-foot pole. I'd guess he risked his life savings with that comment. Hope he enjoyed it. At any rate, with a little persistence and ingenuity, you can still usually get this vital reference check information. Just be certain your staff isn't placing you in jeopardy when they are queried about previous employees of *your* office.

---

## Reference Check

"I will appreciate your helping me to obtain information on __________ ____________________________ who is applying for a position with us. Do you remember her?"

1. When did she work for you? from____________ to ____________
2. She lists her salary as__________________________ . Is that correct?
3. What kind of work did she do? ______________________________
4. Is she a good worker? ______________________________
5. Does she get along well with others? ______________________________
6. What do you think of her? ______________________________
7. What were her strong points? ______________________________
8. What were her weak points? ______________________________
9. Why did she leave? ______________________________
10. Did she have any problems that interfered with her work? Specify: ______________________________
11. Would you rehire her?________ If not, why? ____________________
12. Is there anything else you would like to tell us about her?_________

Comments? ______________________________

---

The key question in any reference check: *would you hire her again?* If they wouldn't, after working with her, do you want to employ her? Review the information you have obtained from your reference checks carefully for inconsistencies with what your applicant has told you. There could exist differences in perceptions concerning some information. Be aware there may also be some deliberate deception discovered. A lie on a factual matter, such as salary level or date of employment, would most likely eliminate that applicant as a candidate.

I believe this final step in our hiring process is critical too. We now invite the remaining applicant or applicants to work a morning (with pay) in our office, and then have the candidate and all staff members of the department they will work in go to lunch at the office's expense. You, doctor, are not invited.

In the half-day spent working in our office, the candidate may find this isn't the place for her. Much better to find out now than three months later, when you get to practice the hiring process all over again! Your staff will allow her to do some simple tasks during this four-hour period, and see if she performs them well, but the main feature we wish to access is ATTITUDE. This is not a part of job training, but the last step in candidate evaluation.

The "free lunch" (remember, there is no free lunch, not here or anywhere else) is the last part of the *hiring process*, but the applicant doesn't know that. The BOSS isn't there, and often the candidate will "let her hair down," having lunch with "just the girls." Twice I have decided not to hire people based on the results of some very candid information obtained during these lunches by my trained staff.

This final staff involvement provides us with one more source of information, but its value is far greater than that. If the candidate's future coworkers say "hire her," *they have made a commitment to her success*. They will work harder to support her, as she is THEIR CHOICE for the position.

I suppose there are many ways to achieve staff support of a new staff member. Such assistance is vital if the most recent member of your team has any hope of being successful. If she is resented and not helped by existing staff, she will fail. Lunch and a half-day's salary is a small price to pay for this commitment. (Obviously this step won't be performed by our new solo doctor, unless you wish to engage the judgement of your spouse at this point—which I would encourage.)

A decision finally reached, the next step is for the senior member of the department to call and "hire" her new team member. Our senior member makes the actual job offer, as she made the hiring decision, along with her fellow department staff . . . remember? All the details of the job are discussed and a date to begin employment is agreed upon. The department can now finalize their plans for training this new associate. A definite schedule that lists the tasks to be taught, who will teach each separate skill and when that training will occur, will be given to our new staff member as soon as she reports for duty.

This carefully planned educational process is even more essential for our staffless solo doctor to perform. It's a lot easier to teach the proper mixing of crown and bridge cement when you're not simultaneously trying to keep a tooth dry. Many resources are in print to help train new assistants. Your ADA Library can again be of service.

With our new team member on board, it's time to send the candidates we interviewed but didn't hire a letter of regret. Be certain before sending these notifications that the person you offered the job has accepted and is eager to begin. These letters are often accompanied by flowers and a personal note of thanks to the one or two applicants that came the closest to being hired.

Remember, even with all the care and effort involved in our hiring system there is no guarantee that the person you select will work out. You may very well find yourself offering a position to one of these people you are now rejecting, possibly in the near future. (I have twice hired people I'd already notified they didn't get the job.) You may also be performing a new patient examination of her soon. In short, you have good reasons to maintain as positive a relationship as possible with the people you interviewed.

## Rejection Letter

Dear

I am very sorry to inform you that you were not selected to fill our current staff vacancy. We had a large number of qualified people apply and only one position to fill. I want to thank you for your time and effort and wish you the best of luck in finding the job you desire and deserve. It was a pleasure meeting with you.

Sincerely,

John A. Wilde and Staff

---

Is this hiring process a lot of work? You bet! Can you take a shortcut and pick and choose the steps you like? I guess. It all depends on your VALUES. How important is the best possible staff to you? Lots of dentists don't have the time for this. Oh, they tell me they would if they made as much money as I. But, if they continue to hire unsuitable staff members, do you think they will ever achieve financial success?

I hope you get the point. Hiring the right staff is a crucial part of the team-building process. I promise, you CANNOT spend too much time or money on any facet of team creation.

Now that you have all the information necessary to hire an outstanding team, ask yourself these questions:

1. Will this outstanding individual, who so closely mirrors our office values, work for the lowest benefit and salary package?
2. Will she accept employment in a rundown and poor-appearing physical facility?

Consistency and values are again the keys. The staff, the office they work in, the way they are treated, the materials and equipment used; all these individual entities must unquestionably reflect your beliefs. *You will not keep great people in a mediocre office.* Don't waste your time trying to hire the best unless you are committed to being the best. Not the Superman of dentists, but a dentist completely committed to become all you can. Use this system to find and hire winners. Then enjoy the success that your efforts have made possible.

## Chapter Thirteen

# Communication and Team Building

In this chapter we'll turn all of our internal efforts—the steps of self-discovery and personal evaluation we've been so involved with to this point—in an outward direction. Through the communication systems that we'll now cover in great detail, our clarified values and goals will be transmitted to our carefully selected staff. The net result of this process is the creation of a **TRUE TEAM** of people, where previously there had existed only a collection of individuals who just happened to work under the same roof.

*A team is a group of people working together toward the attainment of a worthy goal.* I'm sure a book could be and probably has been written as to what a "worthy" goal is. For this discussion's sake, let's define a worthy goal as attempting the achievement of a task consistent with our carefully thought-out values. This prize must be attained without taking advantage of another.

Your team will develop their own unique goals together as part of the team building process that begins with the internalization of the information contained in the following chapters.

A major goal, in the early years of my professional existence, was simply the development of a true team. Once this is accomplished, I believe you'll find both the setting and achieving of more tangible worthy goals an easier task to complete. Tremendous creative energy is released by a group of individuals with one will, now directed by both an inspired leader (you) and a clearly defined mission statement. I can promise you an exciting, successful and fulfilling journey ahead.

A significant portion of this book is devoted to communication and team building. Why bother? You're the intrepid leader and certainly don't need someone to hold your hand on life's journey . . . or do you? What's wrong with giving your staff orders, and if they aren't followed, firing those people and hiring new ones? (I believe making staff walk the plank for disobedience is no longer either popular or legal, also rather unpractical if you practice in a land-locked area.)

Allow me to answer the above query (as I am wont to do) by asking some further questions to stimulate your ability to self-discover the best possible answer for your situation. To you readers with some practice experience, or even you students who can reflect back on your hours of clinical care, I ask: Do you ever feel lonely in your office? Have you ever said (perhaps to your spouse), "It's always all of them against me"? What would it be worth to have not only physical, but emotional support from your staff every day?

The work we do is so difficult. Some patients and procedures make it almost impossible at times. Can you envision working with a group of friends? People who share and understand your dreams and goals, who are there to support you, just as you are there to support them? None of us is an island and no wise man would choose to stand alone. I can't imagine any dentist enjoys practicing in a state of isolation from co-workers.

The proper medication for the painful malady of isolation is an effective office communication system. A mechanism whereby you can accurately share the values and goals you have co-created with your staff. You will become a true office leader, as you now have a destination in mind: the practice of your vision, created through the value clarifying process we have already discussed. With the systems we'll now unveil, this goal can be shared effectively with the people you spend so much time with and who impact your success and happiness so greatly: your staff.

Let's begin by describing the task of a leader. Many of you, by your actions if not your thoughts, consider a leader as someone who gets to be boss, and tells others what to do (if not where to go). This type of leadership is similar to moving a rope by pushing it. Consider the concept for a minute. No one will argue that pushing a rope will move it. The problem lies in control and efficiency of motion.

A true leader is in front, pulling the rope, not behind pushing. The way we get in front as a leader is to:

1. *Create a clear vision* of what your leadership is ultimately attempting to achieve.
2. *Share this vision* with the people around you, to provide them with a sense of direction and to inspire them.
3. Continue to *articulate this vision* at every possible opportunity. Never fall prey to the fallacy that "I've already told them what I think—no need to repeat myself." Do you believe that you can tell your spouse and children that you love them once, and then never need mention it again? Find every creative way you can to illustrate the goals and values that you esteem, and *never stop*.

I would caution you on one point. I think the greater the variety of ways you find to express your vision, the better. Different people will receive understanding and motivation from varied approaches. Fresh and inspiring presentations of your vision will add new energy to your dreams. However, don't ever sacrifice the clarity of your vision for variety. Avoid using analogies that make your feelings less clear just to say things in a different way.

I've frequently described the communication program that exists in our office to other professionals. Be assured, the development of this system is not inexpensive, either in time, effort or money required. The response I often hear is: "I can't afford to take the time that a concept like that will require." Can you afford the loneliness that comes from no one understanding? How much does it cost you to continually have conflict with a staff member (in gut lining, as well as lost efficiency and joy)? What expense is involved when you realize you must fire a member of your staff?

I've often heard it said that to hire and train a new staff member costs $10,000. While I can't prove that figure true, what is the expense of doing a second molar crown prep with your "brand-new" chairside assisting?

I hope these examples help put the investment of time and money an office team building and communication system requires in a different perspective. With a little thought to your own experience, I'm sure you can add a few more dollars as well as frustrations to this total (maybe lost production, decreased collections, messed-up insurance—see what I mean?). I think the potential pitfalls we've just discussed more than justify any expenses occurred in team building, but as a way to ascertain the true value of a communication system, this negative measure of reduced loss doesn't even scratch the surface.

The spirit and creative potential that is generated by a true dental team has to be experienced to be believed. Once an authentic team has been unleashed, the positive effect of the growth of your practice, the joy of working together as a unit, the accelerated flow of new patients attracted by the atmosphere created, and the added productive capability will make all other considerations seem minuscule in comparison.

The series of steps that is our communication system includes three distinct parts:

1. A daily staff meeting and "clearing."
2. A structured communication exercise that all staff must participate in, occurring during our two-hour, biweekly staff meetings.
3. Individual consultations with each staff member, held once per quarter.

Each of these steps is essential to our office's growth and well-being. They were developed separately and slowly in our office and each has value in its own right. It took me years to realize that, combined with a philosophy of practice (physically embodied in our written purpose), the three steps of our communication system had a synergistic quality that multiplied their effectiveness when all are performed together.

I deeply believe these team building ideas to be essential for any practice that desires success and joy. But they are most critical for our beginning solo practice. To escape the morass of debt in which these young heroes so often find themselves mired will require the coordinated efforts of a true team.

## STEP 1: Morning Staff Meeting and Clearing

We have a pretty busy practice. A lot of days I will personally see 40 patients (including hygiene checks). I feel it is essential for me to really KNOW each and every one of these people it is my privilege to care for. We have over 5,000 active patients, and my memory's not *that good*.

I realize a lot of you won't like to hear this, but I get to my office by 6:30 each morning to prepare for our 7:30 staff meeting. I review the FILE of each patient I'm to see that day. I personally make decisions on what x-rays each person needs and note the appropriate films on the schedule. I don't think as DOCTORS we should create and blindly follow generic rules concerning patient treatment, for our personal convenience and at the expense of our clients. I mean standard rules like how often to take x-rays on each patient. Do you really believe a patient that is totally free of any history of dental disease needs the same films as a geriatric patient with active root caries? The frequency and the type of films needed is a *diagnosis* I make for each individual patient, based on my assessment of their own unique dental history.

I also review each patient's record for consistency in treatment recommendations. Do you ever suggest home care, such as a fluoride rinse, and not reinforce that recommendation during each subsequent office visit? Who reviews each record to make sure all previously diagnosed treatment has been completed? (Or does no other dentist pre-authorize treatment and then find at the next recare appointment that it's never been performed?)

How do we **look** when we tell a patient that a crown is needed on one visit, and never mention it again? Do you think the patient doesn't remember? What do you think they believe about our office and how important the care we suggest is? How seriously do you believe they will take our further recommendations, assuming they stay in the practice? (I wonder if I could write a whole book of nothing but questions?) Consider all these examples as they pertain to your desires to develop high-trust patient relationships. Remember that trust may only be earned through our actions.

Are you ever frustrated when all the materials you'll need for a procedure aren't set out in advance? With the complexity of new materials and types of treatment available today, a complete set-up would be difficult to achieve in some situations, even if an assistant were able to read your mind. (A scary thought!) Moments lost when we have to stop treatment to find a needed material or instrument do not add meaning to my life.

Even experienced staff appreciate a written reminder of the exact materials we'll need on difficult or unusual cases, clearly noted on the daily schedule. For example, will the post buildup you're performing at 10 a.m. require Tenure, Fuji II, a Dentatus Post, or some combination of the above?

Almost every day we will experience changes in our patient schedule due to failures or late cancellations. I briefly review the proposed treatment plans for each of our patients scheduled to be seen that day. Since these folks will already be coming to the office, a change in the planned sequence of their care may be the best and easiest way to fill openings in your schedule.

Instead of the two restorations we had scheduled that day, we switch plans to a crown we already have treatment-planned, and our schedule—altered by a late cancellation—is once again filled. Our patient isn't inconvenienced and our staff doesn't have to frantically scramble trying to find someone available on short notice (who usually arrives 20 minutes late anyway). Over the years a lot of hours of productive treatment time have been salvaged in this manner. Since I only see patients a few days a month, I do like to be productive on my office guest appearances!

All these critical items, and many more, I note in writing on each day's schedule. At 7:30 *all the staff are present*. I lead a discussion concerning that day's proposed treatment for each patient. Every member of our staff may have some input.

The front office may add that a particular patient is having a problem with finances. "Please don't do any unscheduled treatment without first checking with us." Hygiene may want us to reinforce flossing, ask how an electronic brush is working, or inquire if more fluoride or Peridex is needed. Some kind soul may remind me of a divorce, an upcoming wedding, a recent vacation, or a loss in the family (and thus reduce for me, at least for the moment, the taste of my own shoe leather). All this information can be exchanged concerning our entire daily schedule, including hygiene, in about 10 minutes.

Do you think this information adds to our production for the day? What does it tell my staff about *my commitment* to our office, and to our patients? How do you feel when the M.D. you've seen for years obviously can't remember who you are? How do you think our increased efficiency due to this preparation changes our patient's perception of the team? Are we seen as caring about them as individuals, not just a set of teeth with an attached wallet?

This review of each patient and his or her proposed treatment is critical, but it's after this is completed that we get to the essential part of our morning meeting: the "clearing." This involves everyone taking perhaps a minute and reading to the rest of us their own current emotional barometer. Maybe today the information they relate is about something wonderful that has happened in their lives.

That's great! After they share this good news with our team, we can all celebrate.

But consider this scenario: All morning long, your chairside is distant and distracted. She fumbles and stumbles. You bite your tongue, until it goes too far. Then you set her straight, and how!

Do you think it would have made a difference in your feelings toward her, and how the day went, if in a morning clearing session, she had shared with you that she had just suffered the loss of a loved one? Maybe it's a sick child or a family member in the hospital that has caused her distraction. Maybe she is ill herself but so loyal to you that she's doing her best to get through the day. Would such knowledge change your perception of reality? I'll leave it to you to put a value on such information.

I feel the greatest value to come from our clearing is this: a demonstration that we all care for and support each other, both as individuals and team members. Maybe today will be a day when **you're** not at your best, doctor. How would it feel to be surrounded by a group of friends who understand and care? Friends who will be there to support you just as you've been there to succor them? What will be the difference in your patient's perception of the team that day? Will they see dissension, or mutual care and support? If you were a patient, which atmosphere would you favor?

An additional benefit of this brief time we spend together is a chance for all of us to get to know each other a little better as people (and not merely fellow workers). Before patients arrive, and our commitment to their care correctly overshadows our personal concerns, we have this time to just be friends and share the good and bad that life brings us all.

Often a staff person's only comment is "I'm clear." That means they are ready to go and able to contribute 100% participation today. Even that bit of information is valuable to know. It's also good to sense that we are all working with friends who really care about us.

This few quiet minutes is also the forum where the team leader (like it or not, that's you, doctor) gets to set the emotional tone for the day. *A grumpy leader at the morning clearing will spend the day with a grumpy staff.* Also, a staff person, perhaps fresh from an argument at home, can have the whole course of the day changed by a few pleasant words here. The power these few minutes exert over the course of your day makes it difficult to overstate the importance of this time.

I'm off the topic, but I have to share this with you. Did you notice that I said at 7:30 all our staff are present? Are all your staff on time . . . always? One person late for a staff meeting is an annoying way for me to begin the day. In the past, when a staff person was tardy, I used to "talk" to them, threaten them, pout . . . you get the picture.

Then a moment of genius! In our office, if you punch in *1 minute* or more late, you are fined $2. The money goes into a "kitty" used to purchase the entire staff's food of choice. (We run strong to doughnuts.)

Anymore, it takes us quite a few weeks to even raise enough "Late Fees" for a dozen doughnuts. We have become an unusually prompt group of individuals. Who enforces this rule? The whole pastry-eating bunch of us, working as a team. (Promptness is a value we all support.) The late and chagrined staff member is now greeted with grateful applause and seen as what they truly are: the bearer of future food! We now *have fun* with what was once a major annoyance that threatened to start our day off in a negative vein.

## STEP 2: Structured Communication Exercise as Part of Our Two-Hour Biweekly Staff Meetings

Our whole office meets every two weeks, at 7:30 on Tuesday morning. The office is locked, with a sign placed on our door stating that we are in conference and will see patients at exactly 9:30. Several chairs are set out in the hallway. If patients arrive a little early they will be comfortable, as well as certain that we are aware of them and concerned with their well-being. (We even set an alarm clock for 9:25, so we never run overtime and break our commitment to our patients.) The answering machine is left on, with a special message saying we will return all calls promptly at 9:30, so nothing will disturb us.

We rotate leadership of staff meetings among all staff, except doctors (we tend to prolixity). A typed agenda has been handed out in advance to each team member, compiled from input all the staff have contributed over the two weeks since our last meeting. A blank agenda form has been posted on the lab wall since the end of our last meeting, to make it convenient to jot down staff meeting ideas during the work day, as they occur to people.

Each agenda item includes the name of the person who wishes to discuss the topic, and how many minutes they request to voice their concern. We time each item with a stopwatch, so we stay on schedule and all topics get the attention needed to properly consider them. Items not on the agenda are discussed at the end of the meeting, time permitting. Of course, staff are paid their normal salary to attend. We don't allow food (not even our beloved doughnuts) in the meeting. This is work!

Chapter Fourteen will be devoted to the staff meeting per se. Our concern here is with the communication segment of the meeting, so if some of the portions of the meeting itself seem sketchy at this point, please don't be concerned, as all your questions relating to details of our staff meeting process will soon be answered.

Now we come to our staff meeting's somewhat unique beginning. It's something we've done for years. **I hate it!** I hate getting ready for it. If it weren't so important to my growth as a person, and our team development, I'd drop it like a hot rock! One more thing . . . **this concept will scare you to death!**

We call it our *communication exercise,* and it consists of two sections: incompletes and positives. Each staff member is REQUIRED to have prepared at least two of each type of communication message to give. There is no maximum number of messages that can be given, but every staff member must be involved, as if nonparticipation was permitted, this whole concept wouldn't last two weeks. As essential to our office growth as this process is, I think you'll soon understand how difficult it is to perform. Sadly, it's tempting to abandon difficult things, even ones you know to be helpful. I believe any smoker or dieter can attest to this fact. That is why complete staff participation is mandated.

We begin with the *incompletes*. This is a statement made by a staff member describing something which happened, that left them with "feelings" that aren't complete. The EXACT situation that occurred (with time, dates and names) is stated, as well as how the event made the person now giving the message feel. All communications given must be carefully prepared in writing before the staff meeting begins. These messages are too sensitive and important for staff to just "wing it."

Once a communication is given, no dialogue is allowed. Such discussions always end up with each party trying to prove that they are "right." (Which implies that someone else is "wrong.") These exercises have nothing to do with right or wrong. They are about a specific event that occurred and how that incident made a staff member feel. Here's an example of an incomplete:

Betsy: "John, when you left Thursday evening before reviewing the last patient's medical history and x-rays, I felt unsupported and concerned about your commitment."

You bet the doctor gets them! The whole idea is open, honest communication. If you allow yourself to get defensive, and explain that you were in a hurry to give blood (and you may have had a NOBLE excuse, but Betsy didn't know that and this is how she felt), any chance for open and honest communication in your office has ended.

Are you scared yet? How many feelings do you think your staff has stored up that they'd like to share with you? Guess who gets the most incompletes? The doctor, at least at first. This trend to doctor incompletes changes, as either the behavior of the doctor evolves, based on the new values and the feedback this system provides, or the entire plan is abandoned as repeated offensive behavior leads to more and more painful communication. Don't begin this system until you are sure your commitment to change and growth is sincere.

So, other than being crazy and masochistic, why would anyone choose to engage in such a process of flagellation? You choose to complete these exercises so you can learn about yourself. You need to see how you are honestly perceived by your staff (and perhaps, your patients?); to show your commitment to growth as an individual and as a team member; to be honestly able to see your actions through another's eye and decide if YOU CHOOSE to change and thus **become close enough to your staff that you can tell each other the truth!**

All have feelings, and we can't control what emotions we have. However, we can make one vital decision: Do we prefer to be honest or dishonest with these feelings? Dishonesty (as in being nice, and not mentioning what upset you, at least not to that person's face) is often easier, or seems so. Until a staff member quits, or goes into a rage. Once again our actions bear witness to the fact that easy is seldom best and that honesty and courage are the superior policies if we wish to thrive.

As I stated earlier, no dialogue is allowed during our communication exercise, with one exception. The staff member giving the communication exercise can make a *request* for a change in the behavior of the staff member to whom the communication is directed. Let's go back to Betsy's incomplete and see how this might work. The request is stated immediately following the incomplete.

Betsy: "John, I request that you stay at the end of the day until all x-rays are read and medical histories have been reviewed."

The person receiving the request now has three options:

1. They can simply say yes. They accept the request and commit in the future to adopt the suggested behavior.

2. They can say "no." We much prefer a candid "no" to making a commitment that will not be kept. Such a failed responsibility just adds to the team's frustration and reduces the staff member's credibility.

3. They can counter-offer, or propose a second alternative.

An example might be:

John: "It's not always possible for me to stay late, Betsy. I will make a commitment to remain in the office when I can, and on evenings when I'm unable to wait, to inform you before we see the last patient, so you will be aware that I have to leave."

The person who made the original request (Betsy) can now say "yes," "no," or counter-offer again. Almost always a solution is arrived at, because we share a common purpose, and are merely seeking the best possible way to achieve this mutual goal. Even in the cases where no agreement can be reached, both parties now understand the other person's situation and point of view. Not infrequently we find the injured feelings were the result of an honest misunderstanding which the communication exercise allows us to clear up.

Allow me to re-emphasize a critical point: No dialogue besides the three choices outlined above is allowed. The rest of the staff is NOT ALLOWED to speak. At the end of a staff meeting, concern about a decision reached can be raised, but the guidelines during the communication exercise itself are strict. If you are lax on these rules prohibiting discussion (and human nature being what it is, people will want to jump in and discuss the topics that are raised), you'll see the system break down to squabbling and self-defense. Neither is compatible with growth.

I believe you can see how consistent with our office philosophy such honest communication is. We accept the short-term discomfort both by sharing our honest feelings and listening as others express theirs. The long-term gain is the creation of a relationship based on openness and honesty that is possible because all the people in our group work in an atmosphere of high trust.

I believe the initiation of this exercise requires great courage from the doctor. You not only have to participate in the exercise, you have to set the example, if you wish to work with **friends**. You must accept the comments given to you in a positive manner, as the potential tools for your personal growth that they are. *Any show of defensiveness on your part will end the honest communication given to you by the staff.* If you want a committed team that pulls together, unselfishly, honesty is the venue by which this is achieved. Did you think a thing of such value would be easy?

The *positives* are easier both to accept and explain. Each staff member recalls at least two things that have occurred which left them with positive feelings toward another staff person. In our office, this is often somebody being thanked for bringing food, but whatever the event was, it's nice to take the time to acknowledge it.

An example here would be:

John: "Betsy, when you stayed into your lunch time to reseat a temporary crown I felt teamed and supported. You showed what a true commitment to our purpose looks like. Thanks!"

I tend to be a critical person. That is my nature, but it's not what I wish to be. For me, the effort to concentrate on the positive in my fellow workers is as essential as anything I do in the office or out. I never have less than four positives to contribute personally (two are required), and am much more likely to have eight.

There is a school of management that talks about how important it is "to catch your people doing something right, and celebrate." We too often practice dentistry in a negative environment. A patient with 31 healthy teeth often hears only of the one other—the tooth with a problem. Here is our chance to celebrate the positive things in life. If you want behavior repeated, REWARD IT! Especially you, doctor—the visionary and leader—must make a determined effort to "accentuate the positive."

The power of these communication sessions, beyond their ability to forge a team of shared value, and encourage individual growth, is that they will lead to changes in individual staff members' behavior.

If I personally take a staff person aside and discuss with them behavior I feel not in the best interest of our team, that is my opinion. If that same staff member is given seven incompletes from seven different team members concerning the identical situation, it is very hard for anyone to ignore such feedback. One of two things will soon occur:

1. The behavior in question will change.
2. The staff member will realize that due to an honest difference in values, our office is not the place for them to be at this time.

### STEP 3: Individual Consultations Between Each Staff Member and the Doctor

We attempt to have these consultations on a quarterly schedule. They probably should be held more often, but of all the communication steps, these are the most time-consuming for the doctor both in terms of preparation and in holding the individual meetings themselves.

Before we sit down together, both the staff member and doctor fill out identical forms, in writing. When we do meet, in a quiet and private setting, we have at least 30 minutes of uninterrupted time available. Our first action is to exchange these already completed forms, and take a moment to read each other's comments.

The first part of the form asks both the doctor and staff person to list separately the activities we feel the staff person is doing extraordinarily well. We share our perceptions of these positive observations. This is a pleasant way for both of us to begin our meeting and often positive contributions are mentioned that the other party hadn't been fully aware of.

The next section of the form instructs us to list *specific goals* which we both feel should be worked on by that staff person. After comparing each other's lists, agreement is reached on one or occasionally two goals we feel need immediate attention. (Don't allow an overly eager staff member to identify more than two goals, or you'll lose the tight focus and concentration needed for meaningful change to occur.) We write these mutually agreed-upon projects on both our copies of the form and each signs them. These "contracts" are placed in the employee's permanent personnel file.

At the next individual consultation, an identical form is filled out before we begin, but previous to exchanging these new documents, we evaluate how the staff person has done concerning the mutually agreed-upon goals from our last meeting. We normally adjust staff salaries every 6 months. Staff people who haven't kept their commitments, as agreed to in writing during these consultations, are not eligible for raises. Of course, the more commitments made and kept the greater the increase in remuneration forthcoming.

Often I get the most value from these individual discussions after the formal meeting part has ended. Despite our years of communication exercises, there remain some topics so delicate that they can only be shared on a one-to-one, closed-door basis. Often I'll hear the same concern expressed by several people. This allows me to deal with a problem (usually involving a specific individual) before I would have even known it existed without this opportunity.

Having performed these practice building exercises for many years, I realize full well the commitment of time, money, effort, and discomfort they represent. (One reason we exchange written ideas in our individual consultations is because I used to fail to address the things I most wanted and needed to discuss, when face to face. My discomfort level, at times, overcame my commitment.)

I hope that the advantages inherent in these systems are readily apparent to you. I would like to caution you to be very patient, yet firm, in working to get your staff involved in this process. Patience is only fair as they have not gone through the value clarification process that you are experiencing. They must first comprehend what your vision is, then see if it is consistent with their personal values.

This is especially true for new staff members in a beginning office.

Initially staff will probably believe that if they ignore all this, the whole thing will go away. How many other "brilliant ideas" have you brought to the office over the years that were eventually abandoned? If you haven't made the critical effort of clarifying your own values before this communication exercise was begun, this will be another concept to "disappear."

All that is required to convince them of your sincerity is a consistent effort on your part. With time, that will banish any doubts.

Those of you with existing practices must accept and be willing to face the fact that you will probably have staff turnover as a result of these policies. The length of time people have been with you has little to do with their acceptance of your vision. You may find that the staff person who has been with you "forever" and whom you can't live without will be the one to leave. Whoever departs will take a lot of their personal as well as office turmoil with them. Turmoil is the broth created when people with varied values attempt to work together.

We've discussed why these staff changes occur and that they are nothing to feel bad about. This is simply a part of the process of people seeking to find an environment consistent with their personal values. Be aware of the fact that even the staff which stay, and are committed to the team vision you have developed, will struggle. I'd strongly recommend sharing all or part of this book to help them during their transition.

Would you give anything to have a supportive, creative team? If you're tired of the way things are in your office and life, here's a formula for dramatic improvement. Like most worthwhile change, this will hurt. Change always does. To me the price is insignificant compared to the value received.

You'll make a lot more money in this "new" office. You'll have many more patients drawn by the positive feelings that are so evident there. (Sad that a positive atmosphere is so rare that it merits such attention.) The habits of open, honest and caring communication will carry over to your relationships with family and friends. But I predict the most significant change will be a renewed interest and joy in your profession . . . a profession of people working together to help others. A team committed to mutual growth, the best possible care for your clients and to having FUN!

To those of you just beginning your dream office and only now hiring your first staff, allow me to extend my congratulations! You may begin your office team with clarified goals and ideal systems in place. You will also have the gift of time required to implement all these valuable strategies. It is so much easier to begin properly than to change existing patterns of behavior.

Make good use of this advantage (admittedly, one of the few you possess). Begin these programs from Day One. Don't delay implementing these essential team building steps for any reason, or you too will be faced with painful change and staff resistance when you later identify the critical need of a true team in your office.

Now let's continue our team building process by considering the entire staff meeting process in detail.

## Chapter Fourteen

# Staff Meetings

I fully realize that staff meetings have existed since dentists had to use foot pedals to supply power to their handpiece. (I'm not that old, I just read about it.) I'd guess there are as many ways to conduct staff meetings as there are dental offices. The differences in the forms of the meetings should exist because both the *objectives* of the staffings and the *collective values* of each team that meets are unique.

I want to describe our staff meetings at length, so you can see exactly how the *particular structure we have adopted is consistent with our values and goals within our office.* As you read this description, please review in your mind how the structure, format, and policies we employ in our staff meetings coincide with what you know of our philosophy. What you should observe is that our meeting's form follows the desired function dictated by our goals.

Staff meetings are the instruments that turn "your" office into "our" office. It is in these meetings that we unleash the *creative potential of the staff as a whole.* We perform these tasks of legerdemain by encouraging the entire staff to become involved in the creative and problem-solving tasks of running the practice. It is during this act of creation that ownership of the office evolves.

Using techniques like brainstorming and piggy-backing (which I'll describe fully later in this chapter) illustrates that the potential achievement of a group of people working together creatively is exponential to what the same individuals working separately could hope to perform.

So, as we proceed with the description of our meetings, please bear in mind:

1. Our staff meetings, in their every form and facet, should consistently mirror our office philosophy.
2. As we labor as a team, ownership of the office (as opposed to its simply being a place of employment) is birthed and nurtured in all the staff. This is a by-product of the creative process. Wouldn't it be great to work with a staff whose every member feels as personally committed to the office goals as you do?
3. Note the creative potential that is unleashed when people united by a common set of values work together to solve mutual problems. Attempt also to be aware of the tenor or mood of the meetings . . . one of trust and enthusiasm. Your office will now do things routinely that you "never thought possible" due to the forces inherent in such synergism.

We have discussed the communication exercise performed in our staff meetings in the previous chapter. No further mention of that vital step of our team development will be included. A few of the staff meeting items noted briefly in Chapter Thirteen will be discussed here again to enable us to now fully flesh out these topics. Also, I'd like this chapter to contain all the information on staff meetings so it can serve as an easy-access reference source with which your office team can work.

Let's begin by looking at a copy of an actual agenda from a past staff meeting in our office. There was nothing noteworthy about this particular meeting. It is merely an example of our typical staff meeting agenda that we'll use as the basis for our discussion.

## Staff Meeting Agenda

Date:
Leader: Kathy
Secretary: Betsy

1. PURPOSE

2. Agreements:
   a) not to subgroup
   b) is everyone safe?

3. Communication Exercises
   A. Incompletes
   B. Positives

4. Requests
   Betsy—assist. scheduled later with John—3 minutes
   Carol—Vacuum—2 minutes
   Carol and Kathy—changes on treatment complete—notes in progress—insurance—2 minutes
   Vickey—x-ray on hygiene schedule—2 minutes
   Carol—charges performed off under wrong doctor—5 minutes
   Carol—emergency patients—scheduled for NP—Pano/fmx not estimated—2 minutes
   John—senior programs in line—2 minutes
   John—policy on charity—stress true expense of the gift—3 minutes
   John—uniforms all set—1 minute
   John—pink card, are we filling one out for everyone who makes financial arrangements—even for a week?—2 minutes
   John—comments on Mitch and Lisa—2 minutes

TARGETS:
   Are all medical histories getting new stickers on them?
   Lowell, are your supper breaks o.k.?
   Are we scheduling Lowell's long op on Monday and Wednesday?
   Are we watching Lowell's schedule on Thur. that we are only scheduling hyg checks after 5:00 p.m.?
   Front office: are we getting pink cards/truth in lending?

5. Agree NOT to Subgroup

Date of next meeting:
Leader: VICKEY
Secretary: KATHY

Here you have an exact reproduction of one of our previous staff meeting agendas—complete with typos, inexact punctuation, misspelling and abbrev. I wanted to reproduce it in this fashion to show it as a working document. Many of the notes contained in this document were jotted down during the course of a busy day, and are in a shorthand that is intelligible only to the writers (and sometimes not even to them). We don't take off points for form, but rather award them on the basis of commitment and creative thought.

The leader of this particular staffing, Kathy, has removed this agenda from the lab wall, where a blank form was hung immediately after the last staffing by that meeting's leader. She has typed this amazingly rough document into the rough (but at least now readable) form you have just reviewed. This agenda is passed out to all staff members on Monday, the day before our conference.

The leadership of the meeting is rotated among all our staff, except doctors (who tend to prolixity, remember?) We based our sequence of leadership on the age of the staff (showing great creativity and ingenuity). You may go by seniority . . . I'd definitely avoid using weight as a method to establish the order of your leaders—but in some fashion, get a sequential list of people, and rotate the chairmanship of the meetings through that list.

The secretary of today's staffing takes notes during the meeting, types them, and passes them out the same day of our conference to all staff. The secretary is simply the leader from our last meeting. (We'd never survive two lists!) The notes are a helpful reminder of exactly what conclusions we reached on each of the topics discussed. They also identify in writing who made what commitments, and by what date any promised task is to be completed. The notes are also useful to help us review and prepare for the next meeting in two weeks.

Our Purpose—its creation and function—has been discussed at length in Chapter Four. It is read out loud before the beginning of each staffing by that meeting's leader. I believe that it sets the proper tone for the endeavor we are about to undertake, by reminding us of the shared beliefs that have brought us together. We all know the Purpose, so why read it? As we discussed earlier, a leader gets a vision, and then REPEATS IT! Our Purpose is the physical and verbal manifestation of our collective vision.

The agreements listed on the agenda are an integral part of our office and the beliefs we share. For our first agreement, we all commit vocally and in turn not to **SUBGROUP**.

Subgrouping is talking about another team member in a negative manner when they are not present. We state out loud that we will refrain from doing this, at the beginning and at the end of each staff meeting. We repeat this twice, one person at a time and out loud, as it is so difficult to avoid talking behind another's back, and also because it is vitally important to our team's success that we do refrain from this most destructive behavior.

There is a second obligation inherent in our commitment not to subgroup. If someone breaks the agreement, and subgroups to me, I agree to take them to the person they need to talk with (i.e., the person they were talking about) and initiate a face-to-face conversation between them. Then something constructive may result from whatever the difficulty was that led to the subgrouping originally.

Say Debbie, our hygienist, comes to me in the lab complaining that she can never find her assistant, Beth, when she needs her. (We use the real names of our staff members here, as none of us is so innocent as to need protecting.) Time is wasted during the search process, patients have to wait, and (probably worst of all) we have an unhappy hygienist. (Remember your Shakespeare, "Hell hath no fury like a waiting hygienist," or some such thing.) This outrage occurs despite a solemn promise from Beth to stay within earshot of Debbie's strident tones.

In my youth I would have met with both these ladies, and rather pedantically lectured and scolded. I would have provided them with a solution to THEIR problem. They would have resented my interference, and the solution wouldn't have worked anyway, as I am neither a hygienist nor an assistant. What do I know about their problems? Except now it would have become MY PROBLEM. I have made it so by my act of attempting to solve it for them. I've taken that monkey off their backs and placed it foursquare on mine. The last thing I need or want is more problems! (Does any of this scenario sound familiar, doctor?)

Today, the new, enlightened (at least "lightened" in the sense of fewer monkeys on my back) John would take Debbie by the hand and take her to wherever Beth was hiding. I'd say, "You two need to talk. Use my office and please do it now." The problem is now in the correct hands to solve it, and the monkey is off my back.

If a problem identified by subgrouping is critical to the office, I may choose to check later and see if or how it was resolved. The conundrum may need to be brought up in a staff meeting for our full group's discussion. However, most subgrouping is of a personal rather than procedural nature, and needs to be solved in private by the parties directly involved.

I can think of no activity more destructive to the team's well-being than subgrouping. It destroys both office morale and interpersonal relationships. Patients are aware of the low-trust atmosphere engendered by such behavior. Somehow the unkind words spoken behind someone's back unfailingly find their way to the individual being besmirched. No positive gain results, but a lot of negative garbage comes from such behavior.

That said, and with our two agreements not to indulge in this pastime, is our office free of such behavior? NO! We are human (most of us at least). This seems a behavior to which, despite our best efforts, we humans are prone. We do often find ourselves stopping in mid-subgroup, as our commitment is recalled. I believe our agreement significantly reduces the amount of this destructive behavior among us.

If we can't stop subgrouping completely, are we hypocritical to keep making this commitment? I don't know about you, but if I gave up everything at which I wasn't perfect, I'd have a lot of time on my hands! Remember, it's the honest effort, not the results, that is most important.

Our second "agreement" consists of the question: *Is everyone safe*? We don't get much response to this query today, but in the early days of our staff meeting, it was frequently answered in the negative.

"Safe" means that you are able to participate in the staffing at a 100% level. Said another way, nothing is blocking you from this goal. If a problem exists that makes you apprehensive (not safe), let's get it out in the open and deal with it before our meeting begins. We can't be a true team unless all of us are completely involved in the meeting.

I'm always delighted when someone isn't safe. It means some staff member is courageously about to broach a difficult, emotional topic. You can trust that this will be a key issue related closely to the growth and overall well-being of the office. If we had no purpose, it would be impossible to reassure a person that we support them in this as yet unnamed poser. As it is, we can promise them that if their subject is consistent with our office purpose, they will indeed have our collective support.

Usually said reassurance—that if their cause is intended to improve the office we will all support it—is the difference between a vital issue being dealt with, and the easier alternative of just not mentioning it. As always, the tougher path leads to growth.

To summarize, someone isn't safe when they feel unable to deal with an important issue during the course of our meeting. We do whatever is needed by that person to make them safe and allow them to proceed. You could call this emotional hand-holding, but the usual reason that someone feels unsafe is that they have had the courage to bring up an important issue none of the rest of us are brave enough to raise.

These agreements are followed by the communication exercise we've covered in the preceding chapter. Note as we go along how consistently the values illuminated by the communication exercise mirror the purpose behind all the other facets of the staff meeting. Can you detect our underlying philosophy within each of the steps involved?

The reading of our office purpose, our agreements, and the completion of our communication exercise is the basic team building portion of our staff meeting. The REQUESTS are the nuts and bolts of each gathering. This is where the process of working together to solve problems to our mutual benefit occurs. This is also where the creative power of many minds working as one is realized.

Don't make an effort to study the actual requests on our agenda. They will mean nothing to you. Do note how many different members of our staff have contributed topics for discussion. This is one small indication of the team concept—all of us with issues to raise important to the whole. Certainly, some people are more instrumental in raising questions than others during any given meeting. That doesn't mean other staff can't be influential in helping solve them. Let's take one example and recreate the process involved in working through that particular problem.

One request states: "John—senior programs in line—2 minutes." This is a request from me for a quick check on the status of the programs we developed for Senior Smile Month that was mentioned a few chapters ago. In a previous meeting the topic of what our office could do to improve the dental health of seniors was raised. Let's use this subject to illustrate the process of **BRAINSTORMING**.

First, we *commit* as a staff to develop a program for seniors. We all agree the topic is consistent with our purpose, and worthy of our efforts. Then the creative brainstorming process begins. One person acts as a secretary and records ideas on a large blackboard, visible to all. Brainstorming involves a quick throwing out of ideas having to do with our selected topic, in this case Senior Smile Month. During this first stage of brainstorming, no criticism or censorship of ideas is allowed. Every concept is simply recorded by our secretary as stated. **PIGGY-BACKING** is encouraged. This is "hopping on" an existing idea with an additional related thought. The more ideas thrown out, no matter how seemingly far-fetched, the greater our creative possibilities.

One of the ideas suggested involved giving a party for seniors. Piggyback ideas would be to have a dance, to wear costumes, to have a drawing for dental health items, and so on. Eventually our creative ideas wane or we decide we have a sufficient number of ideas to proceed.

Now we begin the process of carefully analyzing each suggestion. Both criticism and additional piggy-backing to further develop the original concepts are encouraged. Some ideas, upon critical reflection, are now abandoned. Others seem to have promise. To develop these ideas, specific people are assigned to specific tasks to be completed at (you guessed it) a specific date. These people, assignments and dates are recorded by this meeting's secretary in our staffing notes for later follow-up.

We use only volunteers to work on our varied projects. The people who pursue any ideas need to be committed to their success. This is the concept of ideas having CHAMPIONS to stand up for them, discussed in the outstanding book *In Search of Excellence*. A champion is someone who really believes in a project and will do all in their power to see it succeed. Such determination and dedication to a worthy goal by any of your staff should merit praise and recognition. Remember, if you want behavior repeated, reward it.

At the next staff meeting we will review the information gathered by these champions and begin to make decisions concerning our course of action. Again, as the problems associated with any given project may dictate, volunteers will be assigned to follow up on specific tasks, by specific dates. These dates are selected by the people doing the work, but once determined, we expect them to abide by their self-imposed time commitment.

What if a pledge isn't kept? In such a case, judgment will be required. First, get all the facts. There may have been a reason it was impossible for the person who made the promise to complete the task in a timely manner. But, if the job "just didn't get done," a problem exists. Perhaps the person originally assigned to the task will request another chance and set a new date. The team will have to decide if this is the right person to champion this project. Perhaps additional assistance is needed.

In our office it's very unusual for an assignment not to be completed in a timely fashion. All commitments, the person who made them, and the date THEY CHOSE to have the task completed are recorded on the staff meeting notes, a copy of which is given to every staff member. Failure to keep a promise is a rare, but very serious occurrence for us. If anyone is allowed to not do their share, or if assignments are made and not followed through, soon the entire system will have ceased to exist. Continuity and commitment are the lifeblood of our staff meetings.

I trust this illustration of how one request was dealt with in the venue of a typical staff meeting in our office will be adequate to begin your team on its own process of problem-solving. Once you have formed a team, and identified an issue, I'm sure you'll quickly work out a problem-solving method that will be ideal for your unique needs.

TARGETS are the mechanisms we use to insure the continuity of our staff's efforts. A target is a goal that we had created in a previous meeting. We review targets to make sure we "hit" the goal. Targets are not projects in the development stage, but rather completed ones. We may need to re-access the status of a developed system, or possibly even drop it from future consideration, if we can see no value resulting from our efforts. The champion of each idea will report on its progress, but all of us must consider the status of the undertaking and judge its worthiness.

Wasting valuable staff time on a project with no appreciable payback is avoided as every task is analyzed by the entire staff at each meeting. We want to eliminate dissipating assets by having someone doggedly pursuing a project they believe in, but that less involved people can see is not worth the effort it requires to bring to fruition.

Our next item isn't on the formal agenda. If we have time, after the targets have been checked, we ask people if there are any other topics they wish to discuss. This could be an idea that was thought of too late to be placed on the agenda, or an inspiration that occurred during the course of the staffing. If no time is left, the topic can be noted on the new blank agenda form and placed on our lab wall immediately at the end of this meeting, for discussion at our next staffing.

We now all recommit, verbally and one at a time, not to subgroup.

The last thing we do before adjourning is for each of us to state out loud that we are *clear*. By this we mean nothing remains from our discussions that needs to be said. Someone may wish to briefly thank a fellow team member for his or her efforts during the meeting. A possible misunderstanding may need to be cleared up. Some upset feelings remaining from an earlier topic can be expressed. Several staff members may wish to commit to a short meeting later that day to finalize a topic dealt with during the main meeting. The point of the clearing process is to be certain no loose ends remain at the meeting's conclusion.

We go from these meetings to treat our patients. The atmosphere we leave the staffing with should be one of excitement and a sense of oneness created by our work completed together. Stating that we are clear and thus 100% ready to proceed with our tasks for the day ahead assures that this is the case. Again, I believe it is incumbent on the doctor as the team leader that, no matter what the tenor of the staff meeting, the team leaves with a positive feeling about themselves.

This is the end of our every-two-weeks, full team meeting. There remains to discuss separate staff meetings that take place between just the front office people and just the hygiene staff. These are held once a month and immediately follow the regular staff meeting. They usually last about 40 minutes each.

Holding these department meetings keeps us from having to tie up the entire staff's time with matters that don't directly affect them, but are only relevant to people in particular departments of our office. Issues that do concern the entire staff which are raised at these sub-meetings are simply placed on the agenda for the next regularly scheduled full staff meeting, to be dealt with then by the full team. We began holding departmental meetings years ago when our staff reached seven members. Before that point in our development, issues could be dealt with efficiently with only one staffing.

We have no communication process in either of these department meetings. All the people involved have just left our whole staff meeting, so there is no need to repeat the team building and communication exercises we've all just completed. In the departmental meetings we rotate leaders, just as in the previous meeting, and also have written and timed agenda. This is posted between meetings in a place convenient to the people of these particular departments.

Meeting with only your most direct coworkers, be it front office or hygiene, helps improve relationships for these teams within teams. Topics can be discussed that would be less than comfortable in front of the combined staff. Both hygiene and the front office have their own set of monitors they have developed and keep for their personal information (and to keep me up to date on what is happening in their areas). Their special monitors are reviewed and discussed during these meetings.

In the past, a few meetings were held with just chairsides and doctors. We decided that most of the issues that arise between us could be dealt with on the spot. We can also use our regular staff meeting to discuss chairside-doctor concerns more fully, if need be. My newest chairside has been with us three years. If your situation is different, with new personnel or new procedures being adopted, you may choose to have a staffing between chairsides and doctors on a regular basis. I would base the decision concerning having chairside staff meetings on your assessment of your office need for improved communication and teamwork among these vital members of your staff.

I know the time, effort and expense for all these activities seems staggering, if not downright prohibitive. Let me remind you of our office production goal: HIGH NET. To achieve this requires a committed TEAM effort. I doubt a single doctor—whatever the number of auxiliaries employed—if they don't truly function as a team, could net our goal of $2,000 a day based on his own energy and creative ideas. I certainly couldn't. Even if this were possible, it would be an exhausting, as well as lonely way to exist.

The rewards garnered from these staff meetings should be partly financial, but when you consider the effort involved, and decide whether the reward justifies the expense, don't overlook the much more difficult-to-measure intangibles. The sense of teamwork, honesty and friendship in our working environment has inestimable worth to me. I also deeply believe in the need for each of us to experience growth as individuals and trust our staffings facilitate such personal development. Consider all these facets carefully as you decide on making a commitment of the magnitude needed to create this system and make it work.

The effort required on your part for true team creation will be tremendous. Your commitment to such a system must be long-term. Don't expect either you or your staff to instantly and unanimously grasp all of this information. What starts you on this course, and keeps you motivated, is a set of clearly defined values and goals, first by the team leader, then shared with your developing team in the manner we've just discussed. Without these lucid values, these ideas have no chance of success. With them, financial rewards and the joys of creating and interacting with a committed team await.

## Chapter Fifteen

# The Stopwatch: A Dentist's Best Friend

I bet all of you thought your best friend was your dog. Well, when I'm hunting (which is **every chance I get**, but never often enough), I agree. However, I'd like to attempt to persuade you that in our office, the most valuable instrument we can employ may be a stopwatch!

That's correct, the office MVP is not our beloved high-speed handpiece, with the neat little fiber-optic light, or even our composite curing light (in that lovely shade of blue), or any of the other gadgets so near and dear to our little dental hearts. None of them, valuable as they are, contains so great a potential power to reduce stress, increase income and generally make our lives in the office both more efficient and pleasant as the humble stopwatch.

I know this is outrageous! You love your high-speed handpiece and all the other marvels of dental technology, as well you should. But let me answer your unspoken question with a query of my own. What business that manages to remain extant doesn't know **exactly** how much time each procedure performed requires?

I submit none, with the exception of "modern" medicine. The typical medical practice has the singular distinction of being the least timely industry ever to exist. We aren't talking Swiss watch precision, or German train efficiency in the medical offices I've been forced to frequent! This is certainly not the example dentistry should choose to emulate.

Just how much does the timeliness of other industries affect our lives? Do you care if the fast-food place of your choice cooks the fries for 10 minutes or an hour? I guess, only if you eat them. Do you think automotive companies just sort of fiddle around until a car is manufactured? Does it bother you, just a little, to wait an hour (with your clothes off) to see your friendly physician? Now the telling question: how long does it take you to fabricate a three surface composite restoration, and *how do you know*?

Allow me to share a parable with you. What follows is a true story from the first days a stopwatch became numbered among my best dental friends and allies.

Years ago I heard a speaker discussing the virtues and advantages of timing every dental procedure. This suggestion was based on his assumption that it would be somehow helpful to precisely know such information. But I already knew. If I didn't have times for procedures clearly recorded, how could my staff possibly schedule them? Still, the speaker seemed to believe this timing a worthy enterprise, and I had invested a great deal of both time and money to travel and hear his presentation, so I invested in a stopwatch.

Unlike most new ideas in my office (where I order the materials necessary to implement the shining concept and by the time all the proper equipment has arrived I've forgotten what I wanted it for) we obtained a stopwatch immediately, and actually timed a procedure!

As fate would have it, the first treatment to appear on our schedule was an anterior root canal, a simple one-appointment procedure for which I had historically allotted 60 minutes of my schedule. This had been the time allocated for single canal endodontics since the day I opened my office. At some point, before our first day of seeing patients in my practice, I had *made these times up.*

We began our timing after good anesthetic was obtained and stopped the watch when the one-step endodontic fill with gutta percha was completed, but before we began the restoration. The stopwatch showed 13 minutes had elapsed!

Now, I'm not great at math, but I knew that to be under an hour. Could I really do **four** root canals in the time I had scheduled for one? Could I make four times the income and still remain on schedule? The ten years or so since this experiment took place have answered that query with an emphatic YES!

Well, by now my interest in the stopwatch was peaked (as I hope yours to be). We placed 3"x5" cards in each operatory, with a separate card for every type of dental procedure we performed. Each card was marked on the upper edge with the procedure's title. On these cards we recorded a description of the dental work performed and the time required to complete it. (For example, on our amalgam card would be an entry MOD—18 minutes.) That was all the information required for our purpose.

We didn't measure the time required to administer local anesthetic, but blocked ten minutes (the smallest block of time available in our appointment book) before every procedure requiring the patient be numbed.

The time for anesthetic differs greatly from patient to patient, depending on the number of areas to be anesthetized, apprehension level, and cooperation of the patient, and many other variables. I never rush in administering anesthetic. Painless injections (or as close to that as is physically possible) are critical to an office's success. (Much more on painless injections next chapter.)

It seems this 10-minute average works out well in our office—some patients requiring more time, some less—but the needed times appear to balance out in the course of the day. I do want to make it clear that we didn't measure the time required to give anesthetic, but estimated the time required empirically.

Such an approach may or may not be adequate for your office needs.

My assistant would start the stopwatch the second we began the actual procedure and stop it the instant it was completed. We didn't measure time to seat the patient, clean rooms, or escort the patient to the front office. We have multiple assistants and rooms, so in our office we have a great deal of flexibility in how these important details are handled. If I operated from one chair or with one chairside assistant, I might wish to record operatory preparation and cleanup times also.

For amalgam and composite restorations we worked on a basis of surfaces restored per minute. If we performed an MOD, DO, F, and MO in a total of 40 minutes, that is 8 surfaces restored, or 5 minutes per surface. Thus, when we wished to schedule 6 surfaces of amalgam to be restored, we knew we needed 40 minutes—6 surfaces x 5 minutes per surface, plus 10 minutes for anesthesia. If times didn't figure out to even 10-minute units, *we always rounded numbers up,* as I'm terrified of being rushed. With everything but amalgam and composites, we simply recorded the length of the individual procedures and averaged those times.

It should have taken a week to gather this information. It took us a couple of months. We often forgot to begin timing, stop timing, or forgot about timing completely. When we finally did measure enough treatment to get what I felt were adequate data, I simply averaged out the times for each procedure, dividing total minutes by number of procedures done. These figures were recorded on a little postcard-sized piece of paper we call our scheduling ruler (example at end of chapter). Thus, all the information needed to schedule any treatment we performed in the office was easily accessible from this one small card.

Today we have multiple doctors working in our office, each with an individual scheduling ruler. We appoint from nine computer terminals, so ALL the staff must know exactly how much time is required—not only for each procedure—but for each individual doctor. Without our simple rulers, efficient appointing could be very difficult to achieve consistently and correctly, especially when changes or additions to personnel occur.

The times required for treatment vary greatly from doctor to doctor, as they should. The point of timing is not to work faster, but to schedule care at the ideal pace which allows for performance at the absolute top quality level of which each operator is capable. We are not recording this information in an attempt to increase our speed chairside. We simply desired to know what time is needed for each operator to complete every task to the maximum of their ability.

Before I became friends with my little watch buddy, I would look at the schedule for the upcoming day and know that I would have time to spare or that I was really going to be under a lot of time pressure. I'd know this for a fact, before the day began. I guess this is an example of subconscious awareness, even if we refuse to allow the conscious mind to exactly name the problem. I bet most of you veteran dentists can make such predictions with your schedule now. Such an perception just illustrates that you already know when your scheduling is inaccurate. The question is, *how long will you live with this inefficiency, before_correcting it*?

I'm a hard guy to get along with (as anybody in my office will be happy to attest). It really bugs me to be without a patient. I keep seeing overhead dollars jumping a fence like sheep. But worse than sitting, I HATE to be behind schedule, even by five minutes. I mean I really hate it! With my personality, proper scheduling is vital, if for no better reason than to maintain my staff's sanity. (I'll be the first to admit, the state of my staff's sanity is tenuous, even on a good day. But at least their rush to the sanitariums isn't being accelerated due to poor scheduling, and its subsequent effect on my moods.)

I've included a copy of part of my personal scheduling ruler for you to peruse. Its virtue lies in its simplicity. The times I use are just that: My times. They aren't good or bad—fast or slow. They aren't meant as an example of how your procedures should be scheduled. Your new stopwatch friend will tell you that.

Is it a pain in the rear (pardon the intrusion of complex medical terminology) timing procedures? Yes. Is it worth the trouble? I guess that depends. Would you like to remain on schedule, each and every day? How would your staff and patients feel about that? (Did someone say **shocked**? Shame on you. I believe an office running according to schedule is as critical to success as any one factor in a dental practice can possibly be.) Would it save a little of your stomach lining to not have upset patients and staff—due to your being "a little behind schedule"—to have a normal lunch hour every day, and barring emergencies, to leave on time every night? Would you like to enjoy the income possible from using your skills at their absolute peak of efficiency? If the answer to any of the above questions is yes, you need a stopwatch.

I don't know if this is directly on the topic, but I want to share with you one other scheduling technique that has greatly improved the quality of my life. I schedule a 20-minute coffee break every morning! We rarely run behind schedule, but sometimes a patient arrives late, I have to retake an impression or have trouble with anesthetic. I love having this time to act as a buffer. If we do get behind schedule I know we'll be caught up by the end of my break time.

Usually I have a cup of coffee and a cookie. (I'm perhaps too honest, but it's just one cookie.) I take off my shoes and read the paper or the mail. I don't return calls. This is MY BREAK! Heaven help the staff member whose scheduling causes me to miss this 20 minutes even once. At the end of this respite I brush my teeth and return to my duties, a happier dentist than when I left. I love it! I only wish it hadn't taken me 15 years to think of.

All the aforementioned benefits will occur once you make a commitment to measure your behavior. That's all timing is—a simple measurement of what you're already doing. Think about your feelings looking at the day's schedule. Do you already know intuitively when you have adequate time and when you don't? Now you will have the information needed to get rid of both the slow and the rushed days, forever.

I speak with a lot of dentists. I know of only one other doctor who has ever timed all procedures. Some of the doctors who work with me have chosen not to make the small effort needed to so greatly improve their efficiency. Please let me assure you this may be the most productive time you ever spend as a manager in your office. Nothing I can think of grants such a significant benefit that will continue to bear fruit for years, and at such a small expense in energy and money.

I believe you will find, as I did, greatly reduced stress from being consistently on schedule, a significant increase in income, and a HAPPIER STAFF AND PATIENT GROUP TO SPEND YOUR DAYS WITH. There is only one obstacle. You have to do it! Please don't let your own inertia keep you from this simple task.

## Sample Scheduling Ruler

| | | |
|---|---|---|
| Multiple Amalgams | | 4 min. per surface |
| Multiple Composites | | 6 min. per surface |
| Anterior/Bicuspid Crown Prep | | 50 min. |
| Molar Crown Prep | | 60 min. |
| Seat Crown | | 20 min. |
| ENDODONTICS | 1 Canal | 20 min. |
| | 2 Canals | 30 min. |
| | 3 Canals | 60 min. |

This is just a brief sample of my own personal ruler. Remember that we allow 10 minutes for anesthetic for each procedure where it is required. I believe you can see how all treatment you routinely perform can be easily recorded on a single postcard. The system MUST be simple to be used. All procedures done by an assistant or in hygiene are recorded in a similar manner on each of our scheduling rulers, such as Orthodontic Records . . . 60 minutes, or 4 Sealants . . . 30 minutes.

Please, get that stopwatch today. At your next team meeting share this concept of a more efficient office. Inspire your staff with your vision. (Lunch on time!) Timing your procedures is a simple team exercise that can change the life of every member of your staff for the better.

Timing is even more critical for you doctors new to practice. You will have to time your procedures almost constantly when first beginning private practice, as your speed will develop quickly, once cut free of all the constraints of the dental school system.

Timeliness is imperative to any dentist's chance for success and joy, but even more so to the beginning practitioner, so critically in need of patients. People won't accept waiting today. If you are unable to see them in a timely and prompt manner, they'll simply search for a well-organized office that can.

## Chapter Sixteen

# The Greatest Practice Builder (That No One Talks About)

Over the years I've been taught or shown so many ways to "build" my dental practice (and thus avoid the dreaded "busyness monster"), it's a wonder the walls can hold the patient farrago that's been enticed in. If I become only slightly more behaviorally correct, I'll be in danger of transcendence! And I guess the ideas work—at least I've always been busy.

I've asked patients sincerely and pleasantly to refer their family and friends (we've tried this idea at least). I've exit-interviewed, newslettered, got "on" the patient's level (except for a Vietnamese gentleman who once squatted on the floor—I just don't have the knees). Roses have been sent, flowers given to a favorite patient of the day, special costumes worn on holidays and other "zany" events held. (Funny Hat Day was a hoot, but the Santa suit got very warm, and trying to work in that large, hot, drooping hat . . . forget it!)

My intent isn't to pooh-pooh these fine methods of practice enhancement (well, maybe just a *little* it is), but to focus on a subject much more critical to practice growth, yet one rarely discussed. It's the art of *gentle, profound, and predictable anesthesia.*

The next time *your* teeth are being treated, ask yourself, "Do I want a rose out of the deal? Or would I rather it didn't hurt?"

(If that's a tough question, take your time, but get a response before we go on.)

My admittedly informal survey (I asked my staff) was strongly biased toward *don't hurt*! (However, I have discovered that one of my staff has been way too long between roses!) Ask around and see if most people don't tell you the same thing.

But don't all doctors provide "gentle, profound, and predictable anesthesia"? No, at least not according to some of the patients I see. One sweet lady in her 70's told me, "That's the first shot I've gotten in my life that didn't hurt." (Seventy years is a long time to wait . . . for anything.) Do you think there is a chance she mentioned this event to anyone else? Is it *possible* the people she mentioned it to didn't prefer injections that hurt either? If you have $5 you can get a rose, but a shot that doesn't hurt can be hard to come by.

I believe most doctors really think "my shots don't hurt" (at least not much), but start to *observe* your patients. Do they tense up, close their eyes (or occasionally kick their feet and scream)? All these behaviors could be subtle clues that things aren't as comfortable as you'd hoped. Possibly I'm unique, but I can feel the tension in a patient, and *it doesn't feel good*. Their pulse becomes my pulse and their blood pressure, mine. And you, doctor, get to do this ten times a day. The patient at least only has to put up with it once.

This brings me to a second major point about anesthesia: "gentle, profound, and predictable anesthesia" can save or at least prolong a life . . . yours. Nothing in dentistry is as stressful to me as treating a patient who can "feel it" or even a patient who suspects they may be about to "feel it."

I once traveled 200 miles to watch a noted specialist at work (motivated both to learn from this great man, and to avoid my own patients for a day). During the course of their day, they incised and drained an abscess for an emergency patient. The procedure didn't take long, but she "felt it." When the abscess was opened and the screaming and kicking had stopped, I found myself out in the hall with sweat on my lip and a really bad headache. Thank God I was only watching!

To me, the most amazing part of this whole scenario was the behavior of patients in the reception room—they were still there! Such unhappy occurrences are not good for dentistry, or for the dentist, staff, and patient involved.

So, I hope you'll grant me these two points:

1. Treating patients without profound anesthesia, or hurting them during the injection, is stressful to everybody in the room. It's something we'd like to avoid, if for no other reason than saving wear and tear on our own gastric lining and assorted sphincters.
2. The ability to provide gentle, profound, predictable anesthesia may be the biggest practice builder in existence. (Or lack of this skill may have the biggest negative impact on a practice possible.) My years of clinical experience have allowed me to become acquainted with a lot of people whose *former dentist hurt them*. Most of us don't want to be the next former dentist, so let's explore exactly how to avoid this fate.

Allow me to begin with this disclaimer: I'm no expert on local anesthetic. On the other hand, I do possess a secret weapon. I have the good fortune to be terrified of needles (the sharp, pointy end of same, at least). This has given me an empathy that borders on the supernatural and explains my own selfish reasons (namely personal psychic terror) for trying so diligently not to cause any discomfort when injections are given.

That said, I believe we have two separate subjects to address:

1. *Gentle anesthesia.*
2. *Profound and predictable anesthesia.*

## Gentle

I've often wondered, do my patients love me, or is it my nitrous oxide? I suppose if nitrous oxide sedation were outlawed,

I'd still practice dentistry, but I try not to think about things like that. Nitrous plays such a central role in my war against dental pain that we'll devote the entire next chapter to a detailed discussion of this subject. My next best "gentle" helper is a good topical anesthetic, placed on dried tissue for a few seconds. I've had doctors tell me topicals don't reduce discomfort. It's really very easy to find out. Just give yourself a little local (you big chicken) and use topical on one side and not on the other. There's no reason you should take my word for it, and this experiment should eliminate all doubt as to topical's effectiveness. We use Sultan Topex, but I think most topicals work well. I select them more on the basis of smell and taste, as they all seem to provide adequate topical anesthesia.

I always "wiggle" the tissue vigorously while placing the needle and injecting, especially during mandibular blocks. As I understand it, this concept is part of the "gate" theory of pain. If the nerves are carrying a movement or pressure message to the brain, they can't carry the "ouch" message.

The last point about "gentle" is the most critical: GO SLOWLY. After a while you can gauge the proper injection speed by the patient's reactions. If you go too quickly, you'll feel the patient tense. I've watched lots of dentists give anesthetic and they always inject a lot faster than I. After the injection, they wait for the anesthetic to take effect (and the patient's back to un-arch—"Don't treat them until their butt is back in the chair"—I guess).

It's much better to numb very slowly, and carry on a conversation as you're injecting to help distract the patient. (If you know his wife is having an affair, mentioning it during the injection would be an almost perfect distraction.) It's a little hard at first to find something to talk about at a tension-filled moment like this, but with experience and effort, this conversational distraction can become second nature too. Focusing the patient's mind on **anything** other than the tip of the needle helps.

## Profound and Predictable

Here I'm *really* not an expert, but I'd like to share a few of the little things I do that may help you to achieve complete anesthesia for each of your patients.

1. Occasionally upper molars, especially second and third molars, won't get numb, even for routine operative, without palatal anesthesia. When a couple of buccal infiltrations hasn't been effective, palatal anesthetic usually numbs the tooth almost instantly.

   When giving a palatal, I place topical, push hard over the foramen area with my fingertip for a few seconds, give the anesthetic, and then tell the patient I'm sorry, because it almost always hurts and I really am sorry. I tell the patient I'd rather hurt them this one time than risk their having discomfort every time I touch the tooth.

2. To achieve anesthesia painlessly on the maxillary central incisors, I inject over the canine, wait a minute and then infiltrate over the central I'm going to treat. If you go slowly, this *doesn't hurt* and the patient is usually amazed, as past injections in this sensitive area were so painful (from that "former" guy).

   I clearly recall, as a dental student, numbing a maxillary central incisor as carefully as I could. The tears occasioned by the pain of that injection filled the EARS of my patient. There is no reason for anything like this to occur today with our tiny needles and excellent technique.

3. Mandibular blocks can be the real posers. Here are the techniques I use in the sequence in which they are employed.

   a) I've used the Gow-Gates block routinely for years. It's safer and more comfortable, in my opinion. It's also simple to learn.

   b) Routine mandibular block—If the patient is "jumpy" I may give both the Gow-Gates and conventional block before I even begin a procedure.

c) Buccal and mental infiltration. If I were doing multiple crowns or molar endo on a new patient—or a nervous one—I may use all three of these techniques to begin with. I'm not really recommending that. I know it's a lot of anesthesia and medically may not be the wisest, but I really like my patients to be free of all discomfort. (No one ever says, "I think I was too well anesthetized." If they're not numb enough, they may mention it.)

d) Mandibular Lingual infiltration—this I rarely need—usually just for endo or removal of a lower molar. The lingual bone is much thinner on the mandible than the buccal plate of bone, so infiltration on the lingual is more effective.

e) When all these efforts haven't established complete anesthesia on a tooth scheduled for removal or endo, I use the Ligajet. I choose not to use this on teeth that are to remain vital, and I don't use it until the soft tissue is already numb. In my clumsy hands, the Ligajet seems to be more painful than the conventional syringe. It does, however, almost always give instant anesthetic, even on the toughest of teeth—the sore lower molar. However, the Ligajet is least effective on mandibular molars, especially ones with very long roots.

So, there you have it, a few "diamonds" from the creek bed of my experience. I believe that taking the time to be sincerely concerned about patient comfort—and gentle, profound local anesthetic is certainly only one way in many you can show your commitment—is the "greatest practice builder" and one we should all think and talk about.

For some of you more recent graduates, an increase in skill or technique may be required, but for most experienced doctors, I believe it is only a matter of carefully considering the benefits to them, their practice, and patients that more concern with painless local anesthesia can provide.

For many patients the single biggest concern of any dental appointment, more than fee, convenience, or pleasantness of the staff, is "Will it hurt?" It's very possible for you to look them in the eye and say "No, it will not."

Patients today, at least in Keokuk, seem to take our claim of painless dentistry very seriously. That's great news to the offices that can fulfill their demands, but a death blow to those that can't. Most patients simply won't tolerate being hurt, even a little.

Over the years many patients who have left our practice—usually over our higher fees—have returned after a single experience with a painful injection or a procedure performed without complete anesthesia. Consistently numbing teeth thoroughly and painlessly gives you a tremendous competitive advantage with modern apprehensive and demanding patients.

Sure, it will take a little more time and effort on your part to keep this promise, but if you or a loved one were the patient, wouldn't it be worth it?

## Chapter Seventeen

# Laughing All the Way

We'll continue our discussion of painlessness in dentistry with the in-depth examination of nitrous oxide I promised you in the previous chapter.

Let us be candid. There are times (and for me their names are legion) when dentistry isn't much fun. It isn't fun for the patient, it isn't fun for the dentist or the staff—sometimes the birds outside my office are uptight.

There are a plethora of events and circumstances which conspire to rain unpleasantness on our tooth parade, but I believe we can agree that the two most common and severe storm fronts to rock our small office worlds during patient treatment fall under the general headings of **anxiety and pain.**

Fortunately, we have the capability to greatly subdue our profession's two implacable foes. Dr. Horace Wells unveiled this boon in 1844—shortly before I entered the profession—and it has been undergoing refinement ever since. I refer, of course, to nitrous oxide . . . my old friend laughing gas.

I fancy myself a scientist, so the data which follows will be in the form of a classic pro-con discussion concerning the features, benefits and drawbacks of nitrous. But allow me to advise you, the overriding tenor of my comments will be a paean—a hymn of praise—to the wonders of this fine adjunct to our so difficult profession.

I retain hazy memories of my pre-nitrous days. These experiences occurred during dental school and two years of military service. But nitrous and I began private practice simultaneously in 1974 and we have been compatriots ever since.

As a behavioral adept—as all dentists who desire success must be—I realize it is most efficacious to begin our discussion by detailing the benefits of nitrous. Soon enough, as with all things, we will confront the problems which exist.

As we discussed in detail last chapter, the single most essential ingredient to private practice success is the ability of the dentist to consistently provide quality care with ***COMFORT***. Nothing will keep patients whom you've hurt in your practice. For adult patients, comfort is defined as concern, gentleness and the ability to provide complete, consistent and painless anesthesia. Nitrous is an invaluable ally in the pursuit of these essential goals.

N2O provides both a sedative, or calming, and analgesic, or pain-reducing, effect. Thus nitrous both relaxes patients at the usually anxious moment of injection and elevates their pain threshold. Nitrous, when combined with a good topical, warmed anesthetic solution and a feather-gentle, slower-than-a-glacier injection technique, allows virtually every delivery of local anesthetic to be given painlessly. As a fellow needle-phobic, allow me to once again assure you that, to many of us humans, the availability of painless injections is an **extremely** important issue—of surpassing more intimate concern than the ever-burgeoning national debt or nuclear disarmament.

Some adults prefer not to use nitrous. Others use it only during injections, then ask us to remove it altogether, or to greatly reduce their level of sedation once anesthetic has been given. The majority find they are much more comfortable remaining within the relaxing influence of these soothing gases during their entire dental experience. I'm happy to comply with our patients' every wish, as our objective is to maximize their comfort during the course of our care.

As helpful as nitrous is for adult anesthetic, **it is close to a miracle for the treatment of primary teeth**. I haven't been forced to give local anesthetic to complete restorations on primary teeth for many years, even for deeper fillings.

I vividly recall the first time I used only N2O to restore primary teeth. On that fateful day necessity was indeed the mother of invention. My patient was a tiny, barely two-year-old with classic early baby bottle syndrome caries. I had started N2O and already applied topical. As I sat with syringe in hand, I simply couldn't bring myself to inject the maxillary anterior region on this tiny child. The decay was fairly superficial, so I decided to attempt treatment without anesthetic. (I felt a referral of this 20-pound youngster with multiple caries to be imminent, anyway.) To my amazement, we restored four areas of decay without a whimper or wiggly from our Lilliputian patient. During that experience, my world irrevocably changed, and for the better.

The advantages of not needing local for primary teeth are many and obvious. No one likes injections—not patients, not doctors—no matter how hard we attempt to make them comfortable. The fear of pain and of needles, the terror of a child whose face is "frozen stiff" (we adults know the feeling will eventually leave, but a three-year-old doesn't), the possibilities of lip biting, accidental intravenous injection and overdose, paresthesia—these are all concerns I can live very well without.

Using nitrous alone—with no local anesthetic—primary teeth can be restored without discomfort, and the relaxing sensation is especially pleasant for children. Virtually every child we treat is enthused and enjoys the dental experience. Over the years, many youngsters have expressed disappointment that they had no more decay to be restored!!!! In stark contrast, I've never restored a single permanent tooth where I felt the patient had a wonderful time and regretted needing no additional treatment.

Years ago, the smell of the nasal hoods was objectionable to some kids and presented a barrier to getting them to first use nitrous. The modern scented nasal hoods have eliminated that problem. I ask a child to smell the bubblegum in our magic nose. (My favorite flavor—of many available—for kids.) Just a breath or two and they begin to relax. Modern nose pieces not only come in delicious scents, but are soft, comfortable, well fitting and available in three sizes—so no gas leaks into the patient's eyes and the air we breathe. The best nasal hoods I've found so far, the softest and most pleasant-smelling, come from the ACCUTRON company. You may reach these nitrous specialists by calling 800-531-2221.

At the beginning of treatment, the caregiver must be certain kids are breathing through their nose. Some "sneak" air from the side of their mouth. I remind them to breathe through the bubblegum nose, and sometimes gently lay a finger on their lips to be certain they comply. The nitrous onset is so fast you can begin care within three minutes of the first breath—much quicker than is possible using local anesthetic.

Lest you think I have some unique hypnotic ability which allows me alone to perform these feats of seeming legerdemain, all five dentists who have associated in my office also routinely restore primary teeth without using local anesthetic.

Certainly, nitrous would be invaluable to my office if only for the above stated uses. But N2O just keeps on giving. It eliminates the gag reflex in almost all patients, while retaining the protective cough reflex. Nitrous reduces salivary flow and tongue mobility, making my life decidedly more pleasant. The analgesic effect seems more pronounced on soft tissue, so prophys are much more comfortable. (We have nitrous plumbed to our every operatory, including the two rooms dedicated to hygiene.) Mobile primary teeth can be simply, safely and comfortably removed using just nitrous and topical anesthetic. Uncomfortable, yet not really painful procedures, such as suture removal, dry socket treatment or crown seating, can be done much more pleasantly, and without local, by using N2O.

But it is time to approach the dark side. The grim news: N2O is not a panacea. Certain situations and patients exist where using N2O is contraindicated. There is some debate concerning the safety of using nitrous during pregnancy. I choose to **never** offer it to pregnant patients. I also don't use nitrous on patients with a history of drug or alcohol abuse, fearing the sensation may trigger a renewal of their condition.

If a patient can't breathe through the nose, due to a cold or allergies, nitrous can't help us. (I reschedule kids unable to breathe through the nose rather than treat them with local.) Claustrophobics can't stand to have their nose covered and some people find the N2O sensation to be unpleasant. (Virtually no kids object to the "floaty" feeling.) N2O is contraindicated for patients with chronic obstructive pulmonary diseases, such as emphysema, severe chronic bronchitis and tuberculosis. This entire list of patients for whom N2O isn't available accounts for less than five percent of the people I treat.

There are no known allergies to N2O, and the gas is not irritating to the respiratory system. Because nitrous is not absorbed by the blood, but leaves the body quickly through the lungs, no organ system must break the drug down to excrete it. Most patients feel no lingering effects of N2O after the five minutes of pure oxygen I give them as I complete the last portion of that day's treatment. The most common side effect is nausea and vomiting. This occurs most frequently with children and results from too much gas for too long a time. Dentists need to learn to observe their patient for signs they are too sleepy, then reduce the gas level. I haven't had a patient get sick while on N2O for many years.

I personally begin all kids on five liters of oxygen and four liters of nitrous. On rare occasions, I need to increase the N2O to five liters to get the desired effect, but I never go above the 50% level for any patient. If a child is too sleepy, reducing the nitrous to three liters invariably solves the problem.

I begin most adults on five liters of oxygen and two liters of nitrous. While N2O acts as an analgesic on primary teeth, we are benefiting mostly from the sedative effect on adults (we must still use profound local anesthetic to treat all permanent teeth, no matter what the patient's age), so lower doses are adequate for our purpose. I find the level of nitrous needed to achieve our desired relaxation on adults varies from one to five liters, with 90% of patients feeling maximum comfort between two and three liters. I ask patients to tell me immediately if they feel uncomfortably drowsy and I adjust the N2O level down. If, after two minutes they feel no effect, I increase the nitrous level. Once we have identified their personal comfort zone, I note the ideal N2O dosage on their chart and use that level at every subsequent visit.

Some medical conditions are aided by using nitrous. Room air has a 20.9 percent oxygen concentration. I never give less than 50% oxygen, so for any patient where enhanced oxygen flow is beneficial—such as angina and cardiac sufferers—N2O is helpful. Nitrous acts as a muscle relaxant and reduces the stress of dental care for patients with tender TMJs.

There are concerns about effects on the health of staff members exposed to trace N2O in the operatories. The studies available on this topic are somewhat confusing. Many deal with hospital operating rooms where other gases are used in combination with nitrous. Some dental studies took place without scavengers being part of the systems evaluated. Let me stress that scavengers—which greatly reduce the level of N2O in operatories—should always be a part of any nitrous system. Rooms should be well ventilated, working with a rubber dam reduces N2O leakage, and patients should be limited in their talking—all efforts which reduce trace gas levels within treatment areas.

The medical concerns for staff members exposed frequently to trace amounts of nitrous include reduced fertility, possibly greater chance of spontaneous abortion, and some potential tendency to increased liver and kidney problems. I have re-read all available studies concerning dangers to staff from trace N2O. When used properly, as we've just described, I am not personally concerned about trace nitrous health risks.

Nitrous oxide recreational use and abuse is a problem limited almost entirely to doctors due to their easy access. Prolonged use at very high levels will lead to neurological symptoms akin to those seen with multiple sclerosis. *Nitrous oxide is a drug and should never be used for social reasons.*

The cost of installing a system can also be a barrier to using N2O. A portable unit can be obtained for around $3,000, but I believe those who purchase such a system will find the inconvenience of dragging it around will limit their use. If a plumbed or fixed system is installed, ACCUTRON will lease the flow meter, the main regulator of N2O and major item of expense, for as little as $10 per month.

An operatory can then be totally set up with nitrous for around $700. Often dental meeting specials will allow a system to be purchased at a significant discount, sometimes up to 50%. ACCUTRON seems to make a particularly diligent effort to facilitate the beginning practice's ability to afford an excellent nitrous system.

There are two advantages to nitrous which make it a value to me, at almost any price. The first is the reduction in stress and distress for my patients its use provides. This greatly decreases the tension of providing care for myself (a fragile creature) and my staff. Certainly, the quality of my dental work is enhanced by working on comfortable, relaxed patients with reduced gag reflex, less salivary flow and tongue mobility—and I need all the help I can get! N2O even makes my jokes funny!

The second overwhelming advantage of N2O is in the realm of practice enhancement. I have no objections to those who assess a separate fee to administer N2O, but I don't charge patients who choose to use nitrous. (I'd pay some to use it!) Remember, it isn't your Yellow Pages, direct mail campaign, fancy office or even oh-so-tight margins which build a thriving dental practice. It is your patients telling their friends that "My dentist doesn't hurt me." Creating this reputation within the community is of much greater value to me than any revenue forthcoming from a nitrous fee which would limit its use.

Not only is the ability to offer painless treatment the ultimate practice builder, but nothing can give me greater satisfaction than knowing I was able to provide optimal care in the most comfortable possible manner—especially to children.

I have a dream. It is to live in a world where the words "I hate dentists!" are never spoken. Nitrous is one piece of the puzzle which moves my dream closer to becoming reality.

# Conclusion

So much said, yet so much remains to be told. This is the third book I've written for my fellow dentists and in some ways has proven the most frustrating. I can't ask you kind readers to devote much more of your precious time and energies on my efforts, yet there remain so many additional vital topics of which any beginning dentist needs to be aware.

In these last few moments we have together, allow me to briefly summarize the thoughts I've shared with you to this point and add a few additional concepts for your consideration.

***THE KEY IS CLEAR PERSONAL VALUES!*** I know, I've bludgeoned you with this concept (but you're accustomed to beatings of varied sorts if you survived dental school). I observe so few people of any career persuasion who, by the fruits of their actions, indicate to me the existence of a concisely thought-out master scheme for their own lives. These unclarified people are doomed to be forever adrift, much as a rudderless boat, propelled by the prevailing winds of life in whatever direction these random forces happen to blow at the moment.

Clarified personal values facilitate your creation of a pristine, vibrant life philosophy—as hard and pure as diamonds. This certainty, in turn, allows you to create the intense focus that one must maintain to be successful in these difficult days within our nation in general and profession specifically. Personal energy, applied through the orifice of this narrow focus, provides you with consistent answers to the myriad problems with which career and life will confront you.

If you fail in this most basic endeavor of personal value identification, nothing much I—or anyone else—tells you can have a significant effect on your life or career. You'll be deflected in your course by every bit of advice received from the latest "expert" you've talked to, read or heard speak.

Despite what others may tell you, there is no one right way to live, no one right way to practice our profession. There does exist a best way for you to live and labor, but only you may discover it. In our fear and laziness—seemingly unavoidable portions of the human condition—we continue to peer without for our answers, to search for others to provide the solutions to our problems.

This entire book exists for no other reason than to facilitate your journey **within**. If in some small way I have accomplished that feat, I am a happy man! But be warned, this lifetime internal journey requires fortitude and COURAGE in an amount that few seem to possess.

It is frightening to clearly define your own pathway in life and then steadfastly follow this vision, regardless of the circumstances life confronts us with. It is so much safer to let the ideas of others—our parents, teachers, friends—direct us. When other-guided, if we fail, the onus is on "them." (There exists no such thing as failure, only action and reaction, both of which may guide us, but this concept may take you a lifetime to appreciate. Yet, how sweet is a life with no fear of failing!)

The times you enter are hard, especially if you have chosen to mortgage your future with debt. (And debt is always a **choice**, unless you were coerced at gunpoint to sign loan papers.) Our modern tax codes and other government interference have deeply handicapped our profession. OSHA and its ilk, plus the growing intrusion of third-party plans, are twin cancers, eating away at dentistry's vitality.

Average dental office overhead in 1965 was 45%. In 1975 that figure had risen to 57%. The latest estimate I've seen for 1995 is 68%. To many of you, not yet blooded in private practice, these are mere numbers. To those of us battle-scarred veterans, these are indications of brightly red, pulsating ARTERIAL BLEEDING. Our profession's margin of profitability has been reduced from 55% to 32%—almost cut in half—with no end to this trend in sight.

In plain language, this means today we must produce almost double what was required in 1965 to make the same profit. And this DOESN'T include the pernicious effect of two other steadily growing malignancies—inflation and taxes.

We solo dentists are akin to a deer in the forest fleeing from an entire pack of feral wolves. Our plight reminds me of the line from *The Best Little Whorehouse in Texas*, where the sheriff says he feels like a country dog in the city. If he stands still they screw him, and if he runs they bite him in the butt. Some choice.

Yet, it can be done; financial success and joy are still yours for the taking. No longer is merely opening the door to your office any guarantee of success. Today's conditions demand much more from all of us, neophytes and veterans alike. So, after all the rhetoric, what specifically must we do to achieve the financial independence and happiness we have struggled so hard, merely to be granted the OPPORTUNITY—the POSSIBILITY—to achieve? There are three steps which you must master to reach the golden prize you seek. All are essential parts of the success formula we must achieve if we are to obtain our goal:

## 1. Clinical Excellence

**You must become and remain excellent at the delivery of dental care.** This means you have no choice but to become a perpetual student of dentistry. Upon professional-school graduation, you have learned the basic tools of dentistry and earned the legal right to practice our proud profession. It is now your obligation to transmute these crude instruments into honed and polished SKILLS. The fine sheen of excellence will require many additional years of lucubration to achieve.

Quality continuing education is a must. There are many worthless courses lying in wait for you out there. You must seek the best diligently. As is so often the case, the finest often costs more. Reflect on the time, money and sheer energy you have invested so far in your prodigious efforts. Your drive to learn, now freed from both the constraints and discipline of formal schooling, must never be allowed to languish.

Dental magazines and books can be of great help. Visiting the offices of fellow dentists can prove a wonderful accelerator to the learning process. But most important is your attitude and self-image. See yourself as someone who is always learning—always questing for more. Your office is your laboratory. Focus and work diligently to solve the problems with which your patients will present you. If you but care enough, you'll find the way. But be warned—many never do.

## 2. The Business of Dentistry

You must, from the day your dream of an office is born, see our profession as a business. This essential trait is fragile within our profession. Historically, many decades passed when, due to the shortage of dentists, the poorest of dental businessmen could survive—if not thrive—financially, almost by happenstance. THOSE DAYS ARE NO MORE.

Again, the key is your self-perception. You must rightfully see yourself as the CEO of a small business and carefully analyze each detail of your enterprise. Every facet of your business is your responsibility to monitor. The job never ends.

There are many books, both within and without our profession, that can serve your needs here. Humility aside—if you've found value and meaning in this tome—my first two books will be of great service to you in this quest. I must tell you that about 20% of the material from those first efforts is included, in updated form, within this book. That still leaves you with over 400 pages of new information awaiting.

In my first book, *Bringing Your Practice Into Focus,* my personal philosophy of practice and life is greatly expanded. Also, one-third of the book deals with the very basics of investing at the nuts-and-bolts level (such as what is a bond—municipal, government or corporate—and where and how do you purchase them?). This investment advice is essential information for any beginning practitioner who has dreams of financial success.

My second book, *How Dentistry Can Be a Joyous Path to Financial Freedom*, again touches on philosophy, has a solid section on management and marketing, and goes into greater depth concerning investment concepts. In this book I have created a matrix of financial choices that will identify the ideal investment for each individual at any point in your career, and explains the details of how the appropriate transactions can be accomplished. I believe this information to be **invaluable** to anyone who dreams of financial independence.

Both books can be ordered by calling 319-524-8811 or faxing 319-524-9785.

I'm sorry to admit this book—due to space constraints—hasn't given the emphasis to debt reduction and money management that forms a vital part of any individual's chance to obtain financial freedom. I'm delighted to tell you this critical information is available in my other books.

## 3. People Skills

As is the case with business skills, you have had virtually no training in the art of dealing with people. A lot of *How Dentistry Can Be a Joyous Path to Financial Freedom* focuses on this critical subject, and mastering it is essential to your success. If you open an office and do everything I've discussed to date perfectly—but possess no behavioral skills—you are doomed.

There are many resources available to help you become behaviorally adept. Thousands of books have been written on the subject. The mere number of literary efforts in this venue attests to how essential these skills are to every form of endeavor. Among those that have most influenced my career and search for joy are:

*Think and Grow Rich*, by Napoleon Hill
*Psycho-Cybernetics*, by Maxwell Maltz, M.D.
*In Search of Excellence*, by Thomas Peters and Robert Waterman
*The Seven Habits of Highly Effective People*, by Stephen Covey

Each of these classics should be available from any bookstore or library. These are texts I've read, reread, underlined, taken notes on and then picked up again years later. I've studied hundreds more, but this is more than a full plate for you now, and represents the true cream of the genera, in my opinion.

Do you comprehend that to understand others you must first understand yourself? To reach your ultimate potential as a health care provider, you must truly become a person who cares for others—family, friends, staff, patients and maybe someday your fellow man. I know of no tricks to help you. The road to success behaviorally is self-understanding and self-love that will reflect out to the world around you. This great achievement must be earned.

Above all, never lose sight of the ultimate goal. It is not wealth and all the wonder it can provide. Not a good reputation or people who care about you. It is simply the attainment of JOY. Achieve that central goal and everything you long for will be yours. Fail to achieve joy, and the sweetest of fruits will taste of bitter ashes. Reflect back on our first chapter together entitled "The Subject Was Joy." If your life isn't moving toward ever-increasing joy, nothing else matters.

I wish you the very best. You are welcome to visit my office or call me at home any evening by dialing 217-847-2816, if I may somehow serve you. And may God bless.

# Index

**Note to the reader:** Some topics are not independently listed because they are related to a specific main heading. If at first you do not find what you need, try subtopics under the following main headings: Practice, group. Practice, locating. Practice, purchasing. Practice, solo. Staff. Staff meetings.

## B



## C



## D

# E



# F



# G



# H



# I

# P

# Give the Gift of *The Dental Practice of Your Dreams* to Your Friends and Colleagues

❑ **YES,** I want ______ copies of *How To Create the Dental Practice of Your Dreams* at $46.90 each, plus $5 shipping per book (Illinois residents please add $2.93 state sales tax per book).

❑ **YES,** I want ______ copies of *How Dentistry Can Be a Joyous Path to Financial Freedom* at $[illegible] each, plus $5 shipping per book (Illinois residents please add $2.93 state sales tax per book).

❑ **YES,** I want ______ copies of *Bringing Your Practice Into Focus* at $40.95 each, plus $5 shipping per book (Illinois residents please add $2.56 state sales tax per book).

❑ **YES,** I am interested in having Dr. John Wilde speak or give a seminar to my company, association, school, or organization. Please send information.

Canadian orders must be accompanied by a postal money order in U.S. funds. Allow 15 days for delivery.

My check or money order for $__________ is enclosed.

Please charge my ❑ Visa ❑ MasterCard

Name______________________________________Phone____________________

Organization ________________________________________________________

Address ____________________________________________________________

City/State/Zip ______________________________________________________

Card # ____________________________________ Exp. Date _____________

Signature ___________________________________________________________

Please make your check payable and return to:

**The Novel Pen**
210 Windy Hills
Hamilton, IL 62341

**Call your credit card order to: [illegible]3**
**or fax: 319-524-9785**